LESBIAN MARRIAGE

A *SEX* SURVIVAL KIT

LESBIAN MARRIAGE
A *SEX* SURVIVAL KIT

**KIM CHERNIN &
RENATE STENDHAL**

LESBIAN MARRIAGE: A SEX SURVIVAL KIT

www.lesbiansexsurvival.com

ISBN: 978-0615992365

This book is dedicated to our California sisters and brothers who regained the right to same-sex marriage in June 2013.

PRAISE FOR RENATE STENDHAL AND KIM CHERNIN

FOR *TRUE SECRETS OF LESBIAN DESIRE* BY RENATE STENDHAL (*LOVE'S LEARNING PLACE*, IN HARDCOVER):

"Renate Stendhal shows us, reassuringly and lovingly, how cultivating radical honesty – about who we are, where we've been, what we want, and how we want it – gives us the tools to start creating the relationships and sex lives we really want without starting over from scratch."
–HANNE BLANK, AUTHOR OF *BIG BIG LOVE: A SOURCEBOOK ON SEX FOR PEOPLE OF SIZE AND THOSE WHO LOVE THEM*

"This lovely book offers sound advice on how to relate with one's lover. Its emotionally honest tone posits that trust and truth are keys to unlocking long-term erotic pleasure. Stendhal is playful, practical, and philosophical. She is a warm teacher whose wisdom belongs in the life of every lesbian stuck on the myth of the lesbian bed death."
–RICHARD LABONTE, *BOOKMARKS*, Q-SYNDICATE

"A few self-help books tackle women's issues with a more politicized lens and increased sensitivity. True Secrets examines women's long-term relationships and asserts that truth telling as political act can create a deeper love and is the healthiest, 'least costly,' and most effective strategy available."
–NICOLE BRAUN, *FOREWORD*

"Stendhal is onto something. *True Secrets* is the start of serious dialogue on lesbian relationships, emphasizing their validity and showing that, like any other relationship, they are worth waiting for."
–Jano, Lambda Book Report

"This book is a welcome addition to the small number of lesbian self-help psychology books on the market. Using examples of couple interaction in therapy sessions, Stendhal cites cases from her practice in which self-awareness was achieved. She takes special aim at the shame some women experience around sex."
–Sonja Franeta, The Gay and Lesbian Review

FOR *THE FLAME BEARERS* BY KIM CHERNIN

"Full of surprise and suspense… The richness of traditional knowledge that shines on every page gives the book its depth and humor."
–Anne Roiphe, New York Times Book Review

"Immensely compelling … lyrical … Chernin provides a dreamlike setting for events, a quality found in the works of Gabriel Garcia Marquez and Isaac Bashevis Singer."
–The San Francisco Chronicle

"Worshippers of the Mother will welcome Chernin's bold first novel … The flashback parts are told by the old woman in a voice as engaging as those in Isaac Bashevis Singer's tales of villages, bathhouses, and possession … In all, Chernin keeps us interested through her energetic recreation of the past."
–Kirkus Review

"Certainly women have been reading books, from Scripture to the novels of Philip Roth, in which they play the supporting role while God talks with the men. The Flame Bearers will be read with delight by those who enjoy good ideological revenge, a turning of the tables."
–New York Times Book Review

FOR IN MY MOTHER'S HOUSE BY KIM CHERNIN

"What a fascinating, rich, beautiful book: an illumination of our times – humanly, politically – interwoven with a profound portrayal of the ever-changing, deepening relationship between mother, daughter, and eventually granddaughter. A book that will be an American resource."
–Tillie Olsen

"In My Mother's House adds a triumphant dimension to the body of [mother-daughter] literature. Triumphant not only because it is profoundly moving and splendidly written, but also because Rose and Kim Chernin achieve a rare level of communication and understanding."
–Ann Martin-Leff, New Directions for Women

TABLE OF CONTENTS

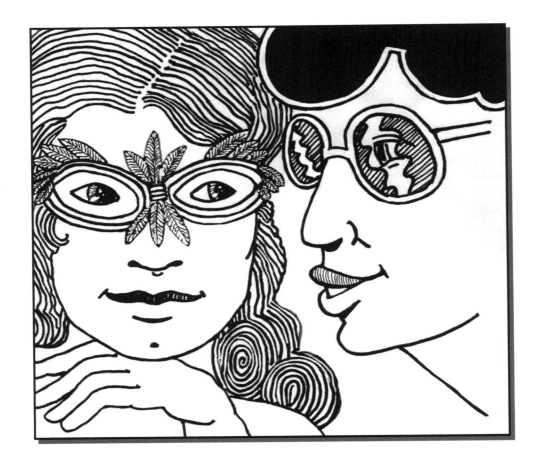

WHAT IS SEX?

WANTED: THE KIND OF SEX THAT DEEPENS INTIMACY AND NEVER FADES.

You care about your marriage; you want to keep your love alive and passionate. If you are on the path to marriage, you want to make sure your sexual attraction won't be lost. Now that you can, you would like to receive all the blessings of marriage – sex and romance, closeness and tenderness, honesty and harmony… until death do you part.

We all know that keeping sex and romance alive is not a piece of cake. Let this book help you along in the spirit of frankness and humor. You will find stories, reflections, and sex survival tools. You will find more than everything you always wanted to know about sex in lesbian marriage.

Sex is…a many-splendored thing.

It's also a trickster: it flares up, slips away, gets fixed on the one and only, changes partners, goes wild, thrives on intimacy, gets going only with strangers, falls asleep, changes form, gets bored, and sparks into life again. When we fall in love, we want sex to be around forever, for better or worse. And why not? We "only" have to figure out ways to release this wily genie from its bottle – again and all over again. Let's have a go at it.

We are offering you a tool kit, handy advice on how to keep sex alive and well. Our toolkit suggests what to do and what pitfalls to avoid when you are in a life-long commitment or headed into marriage. But don't fear, this is not another manual about the 499 Kama sutra positions or 365 daily tantric exercises; it's not glossy magazine hype about guaranteed and never-ending orgasm, or an android app to track your sex performance.

We are asking you to think, to be honest, to look at yourself with a smile, to smoke out the trouble-makers that interfere with your sexual intimacy and fulfillment. And above all, we hope you will have a good laugh now and then.

SO, TO GET GOING: WHAT IS SEX?

- A great mystery
- a portal to the divine
- the spice of married life
- slow in coming
- a pain in the butt
- a pressure cooker
- a way of letting off steam
- elusive nirvana
- the greatest story ever sold
- dreaded obsession
- the meaning of life
- what you're too tired to desire
- the hottest intimacy
- a yawn
- what you have to put up with

- pleasure surpassing pleasure
- unending frustration
- a shameful sin
- a torment that knows no end
- a meeting of souls through the body
- a dream come true

Here's a game to play with your partner while you're waiting in line to tie the knot (a sexy image of marriage if there ever was one).

SEX IS: (FILL IN THE BLANKS)

- _____
- _____
- _____
- _____

Notes, Scribbles, Doodles

INSTRUCTION GUIDE

FOR THE TOOLKIT

As you read through this book, you will find twelve chapters. Each starts with a story we call a Challenge. Each Challenge is then discussed in a section called Let's See. Finally, a list of Do's and Don'ts suggests tools you can use to navigate these Challenges. We'd like to inspire you to take concrete steps to make your marriage everything you want it to be. We trust that this book will help you keep love, passion, and intimacy alive.

CHALLENGE

What we call Challenges are problems couples encounter in all long-term relationships and marriage.

We chose a number of typical, "classical" areas of discontent that hinder closeness, sexual happiness, and aliveness. Marriage brings its own heightening to these trouble-spots, deserving particular attention and care.

Now that lesbian couples are stepping into full recognition by culture and society, there is more pressure to succeed as a couple – and potentially as a family. There is the invitation, as freshly married lesbians, to fill the age-old institution with a new spirit and new forms of living. Our Sex Survival Kit helps you pinpoint twelve all-too-human couple predicaments and offers you tools to handle or avoid them. We have listened to friends and clients of all ages, colors, and backgrounds telling us their relationship and marriage stories. Several of them appear in this book, together with a couple of our own.

LET'S SEE...

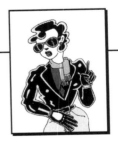

Each of the twelve major CHALLENGES is contained in a story, followed by some reflections called LET'S SEE.

This section is not meant to proclaim The Truth. It's not about big rules or laws of engagement written in stone. LET'S SEE is a way of looking at difficulties with common sense and humor. We bring in our own couple's perspective, having faced the same issues in our life together.

TOOLKIT

The toolkit is a grab-bag of handy DO'S and DON'T'S, practical things to practice doing and not doing. You don't even have to read the stories to make use of these tools. You KNOW the stories! Don't feel pressured to open your toolkit and take out every tool we are laying out here. When you need to put a screw in the wall, you don't pull out your hammer. You know which tool will do the job. The same applies to our toolkit.

Detect the smile in the Do's and Don'ts and the invitation to be forgiving to yourself and your partner. There's humor here even in the very number of tools offered for every problem. You won't ever have to use the whole bunch. After all, how many tools does it take to screw in a light bulb? You might have fun reading the Do's and Don'ts aloud to each other in the bathtub. Be creative and add your own tools to this handy kit.

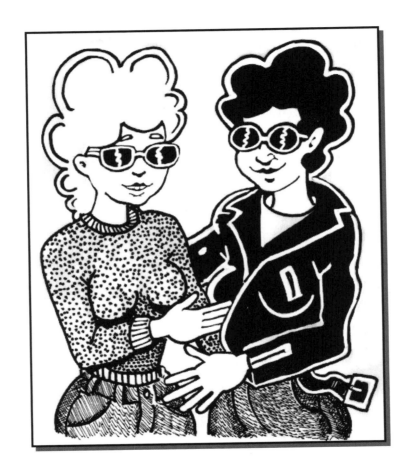

YES, I DO

A DIALOGUE – KIM AND RENATE

Personally and politically, we live in an exciting historical moment, celebrating a dramatic change in the cultural climate. The freedom for lesbian and gay people to marry brings with it unlimited potential and new demands. We wrote this toolkit because in our long relationship "we've seen it all." We have talked to many other women professionally and personally, as mentors and as practitioners of a different kind of listening: a form of common sense conversation. (Common sense because over the years we have realized that common sense is the least common kind of sense.) We have also published several books about women's lives, spirituality, and sex (see our book pages in the back).

We started this book with a conversation. Over a latte and a double espresso at our favorite café, we talked about our personal history of marriage. To our surprise, after all our years together, we learned a few things about each other we didn't know.

KIM: I never wanted to get married. Not ever, even when I was a small girl. I've been married twice to partners I loved and I thought I would live with for the rest of my life, but the marriages were purely pragmatic. The first time, at eighteen and twenty-one, we wanted to go to Europe; we asked our relatives to give us money instead of presents if we got married. The relatives were encouraging; we got married and took off for four years in Europe. The second time, much later, when I was in my thirties, the issue was still financial; it was taxes this time, and we agreed we would not tell any of our friends we'd gone to Mexico to get married. We preferred our bohemian life-style and did not want to be seen as caving in to a bourgeois institution. Two marriages, two divorces, and I still never wanted to get married. As a teenager, I liked the idea of being someone's mistress. I don't know where this idea came from, but I sensed the freedom in it, the independence, the possibility of being my own woman and living a life of my own choosing. No children, no family, traveling a lot, and having as much sex as possible. To my mind, marriage and sex did not easily fit together. I saw sex as something wild and untamed and seemed to know it wouldn't be around for long in a marriage.

So, now, suddenly, after all these years, we are thinking about getting married?

RENATE: I, too, got married very young and experienced a complete failure. Especially sexually. The romantic pressure of succeeding in marriage turned everything into a performance: fake orgasms were the rule of the day. After coming out in my early twenties, I had several committed long-term relationships that were very much like marriages. I loved my partner, did my best, but after the honeymoon phase sex became problematic and slowly disappeared. I concluded that any relationship that was like a marriage was sexually doomed. Marriage was best avoided. I didn't know yet that the problem was miscommunication between me and my lovers,

that some of the discontent might have been worked out in truthful conversation. But there was a basic limitation to these relationships. The women I chose were fine people, but they were not my soul-mates.

KIM: Both of us have been looking for the soul-mate, chasing the twin myth, looking for the matching half of us living on the other side of the world. I already had this fantasy when I was a child, but there was not yet anything sexual in it. Back then it meant someone who liked all the same things I did, like playing baseball and riding bikes. A true soul connection for a ten-year-old.

RENATE: I lived in Paris; Kim was a visitor. We were both writers and had picked the same café out of hundreds of cafés to write in. That's how we met, in a café across from the Luxembourg. I was 38 and had given up on committed relationships. I was polygamous and chasing down sex as much as possible. Nevertheless, I secretly yearned for the woman who would be the true romantic love object and with whom sex would never die!

KIM: I remember walking down the street with Renate and some other women, glancing to my left, seeing her in her long scarf and cap, exuberantly walking along as if she feared nothing life might bring to her. My spontaneous thought was: here she is; my life companion

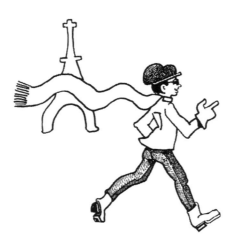

RENATE: I had to give up four lovers and my whole European life to come to Berkeley to be with Kim.

KIM: It took a long time, so many expensive phone calls, sometimes lasting four hours, to convince her that monogamy, romance, and sex did not have to be incompatible.

RENATE: Finally, what convinced me was that anyone who could argue for hours on behalf of enduring monogamous sex knew something I didn't. It made me curious. I decided to move to Berkeley but not to stay one day longer than my passion lasted. On one occasion, I felt I had to return to Paris for business, but I was missing Kim so much I got on a plane back the next day. I knew by then that the problems between us could be worked out because of the way we talked together. We were both language nuts, loving to spell out everything, finding ways to tell each other the truth. That sealed it.

KIM: After Renate moved to Berkeley we wrote our first book together, *Sex and Other Sacred Games* (available on Amazon) Our protagonists were two very different women who finally manage to understand each other by taking the risk of radical honesty.

RENATE: It was clear that we belonged together, no matter what problems we would have to face. We would work it out with honesty and empathy. Telling each other the truth in daring as well as caring ways turned out to be a phenomenal aphrodisiac, always renewing our intimate bond. This was such a big discovery that I wrote *True Secrets of Lesbian Desire: Keeping Sex Alive in Long-Term Relationships* (available on Amazon) on that theme. So, I could say we have felt married all along without thinking about it in these terms.

KIM: In fact, we already married, in a purely private ceremony in a natural hot spring in New Mexico, on one of our recurrent pre-marital honeymoon trips.

RENATE: We had been looking for hot springs in the area and one day climbed down a rocky, precarious path to the Colorado River. The spring rushed forth a few steps above the river, pooling in several natural basins like little hot tubs. At the lowest level, right next to the riverbed, a larger pool had the perfect temperature. We slid in without clothes. There wasn't a soul around, only the majestic river slowly rolling past us. Swarms of swallows chasing over the water and up the cliffs on the opposite bank. We felt submerged in the warmth of earth, water, air, sky, and the strange beauty of this blessing. When we found words, they were a pledge we made of ourselves to the universe and our togetherness. We knew this moment was our wedding.

KIM: When gay marriage was suddenly allowed in San Francisco we were wondering, how is the

State of California going to offer us anything as magical as that? We saw our expression of gratitude to whatever had brought us together as a ritual. We saw no need to make further promises or vows or pledges. We were grateful, overflowing with gratitude; that's what we whispered in the hot water next to the river. And now we're thinking about letting the state confer whatever legitimacy it has to offer? As if our own ceremony was not sufficiently expressive and binding?

RENATE: Although, I always had a thing about weddings. As a child, and all through my life really, I thought there was nothing on earth more romantic than this ritual of giving over one's self to the loved one. A ritual in front of a community of loving spirits, family, friends--if only it could be done between true equals! As a teenager I used to make obsessive drawings of brides and designed a zillion wedding dresses...

Kim: It's really funny when you come down to it. When I was a teenager I was dreaming of being someone's mistress while Renate was designing wedding dresses for herself.

RENATE: I hankered for the impossible--the bohemian marriage of outsiders who wouldn't get trapped and caught in the boredom of convention, what I called the "marriage coffin." When gay marriage became legal I remained skeptical that the institution of marriage would ever be for the two of us. I see myself changing my mind.

KIM: I know what the change is for me. Since the Supreme Court made marriage between gay people legal in California, something bigger than our personal inclinations is afoot. We don't imagine marriage will have any influence on the way we love or are intimate. In our small social world, no one cares if we are married or are two women living together. At our age (old, older) we're not planning to have children. We have one daughter from my first marriage who is living in Peru and finds the idea of our getting married hysterically funny. After all, she's known us as a couple her entire adult life. It probably never crossed her mind that we weren't "married."

RENATE: So why ARE we thinking about getting married?

KIM: Because it has become political. The personal IS political as we've been saying for a long time. I have never come across a more telling example. It has also become historical, and I want to be part of one of the most significant legal decisions that has been announced during my lifetime. When I was sixteen I heard about Brown vs. Board of Education, the Supreme Court decision that required schools to be integrated. To me, the Supreme Court recognizing the rights of gay people to be married is as big as that. Or rather, since they haven't gone all the way yet,

recognizing the right of the states to make that decision, as our State of California has.

RENATE: I think you're forgetting the many crucial battles for women's rights, ERA, free abortion, equal pay for equal work, the victorious battles against rape and sexual harassment, child abuse, and rape in marriage. I could go on and on! Those are just as big for me as civil rights.

KIM: Can't you just imagine the argument we would have had twenty years ago? Some shouting, some table slapping, some storming out of the room. As if the fight for civil rights was more significant than feminist issues or vice versa? Back then we couldn't see both points of view; we felt compelled to convince each other. Each one of us had to be right, as if our opinions were a matter of life and death.

RENATE: Nowadays, we see this pattern between us, our hot-headed differences. Now it makes us laugh. We crack a joke and put the argument in the "dumpster." We already know what each of us is going to say, so why bother opining?

KIM: We certainly agree about sex and gay marriage, and I'm pretty sure I won't have to be on the phone for four hours.

RENATE: I remember the joy and exuberance of the feminist movement, the incredible rights and freedoms we took, and most of all the erotic freedoms. The permission to love and make love without guilt and shame. The generous capacity to see every woman as a potential lover, a person worthy of our intimate attention and passion. The freedom to rebel against any restriction of our desire, to transgress gender, be androgynous, take on any role we wanted, and to redefine and recreate ourselves from head to toe.

KIM: After all, feminism and gay liberation are the godparents to legalized gay marriage. They're going to be right up there at the altar giving away the brides and grooms. I'm moved to tears every time I see how much the right to marry means to people in our community. It's made me bigger than myself, forced my capacity for empathy to expand. I see why my gay friends have been so upset when their brothers and sisters are given huge marriage celebrations by their families while their long-term, enduring relationships are ignored. Since I never cared much for marriage I thought, "What's the big deal? " But of course it was a big deal not to be recognized, to feel excluded from what the family takes seriously. In some situations, the grandchildren were considered illegitimate by their own grandparents who refused to see them. We all know stories like that. When I see myself as part of this larger community of shared purpose, my understanding grows and I want to participate.

RENATE: I feel again what I felt during the years I lived in Paris, the sheer intoxication of a community turning into a movement and changing the world.

KIM: That's one advantage, getting there this late. We're not afraid of the pitfalls of marriage. We've survived them. Think of the cartoon on our refrigerator door, the two very old women in their rocking chairs. One says to the other: "They say, as you get older you get wiser." The other responds: "In that case you must be a genius by now."

RENATE: At least we've acquired some tools for when the going gets rough. And it does, dear friends, it certainly does…

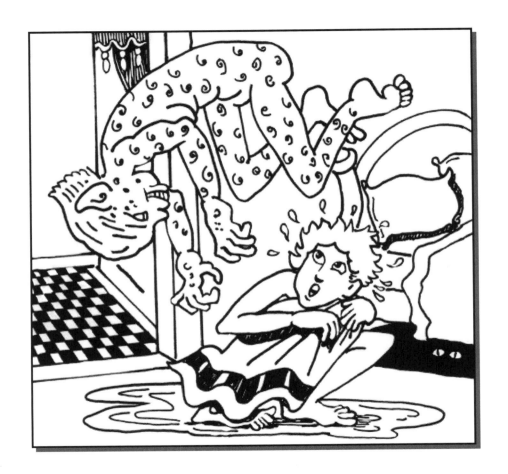

CHALLENGE 1

BUTCH AND FEMME – THE HABIT OF ROLES

This story was co-written by Kim and Renate with permission to quote two of their friends

We decided to do something daring: to meet with two other lesbian couples and talk about intimacy in our relationships. Ask a few questions. Do you still have sex? Are both of you satisfied with your sex life? What are you missing, if anything?

At first, everyone was giggling. One rose up to make coffee, another was checking her email. Another one was going to the bathroom a lot. It took a couple of meetings to get going and overcome the shyness we all shared.

We found out that our six-some had no problem with the O-Word. A challenge, however, for most of us was the question of roles. Each couple had stories about roles. How butch and femme, and active and passive role divisions were "encrusted" and tricky to change, no matter how much we'd like them to be different. Who initiates and who doesn't, who makes love to whom and does it well,

took a lot of room in our talks and pretty soon we were talking about nothing else.

One of the most typical stories that emerged was told by two of our friends who had been together for eight years and were getting ready to tie the knot. Maria was born in Rio, Brazil and was a teacher of African dance. She was three years older than Lee, a researcher in the field of education, who had grown up in Skagway, Alaska. They had met online, and their attraction was initially based on the sun and ice of their different backgrounds. Lee had moved to San Francisco to be with Maria. They were both living far from home but felt their love bond made up for the distance from their families who would never have approved of their relationship. The two of them were each other's home.

MARIA: "For about three years, we were like two chameleons who could easily change color and play with fantasies. But it was always the same role division. I was the top. We had a great time with it. I would be the Brazilian fairy-tale toad, leaping onto Lee who was the meek little lamb; or I would play the Alaskan hunter and Lee the seal pup that gets hunted down and eaten up. We sometimes used a few disguises; for example, I put on a fur collar to be the bold, irresistible hunter, and Lee would squeal with delight when I came after her. I thought I was really a dynamite butch, the best lover on earth, to tell you the truth. But maybe it was also that Lee was such a gifted femme that I just couldn't go wrong with her. She simply found everything a huge turn-on. So we thought we were a real success in our sex life. Until one day it didn't work any more."

LEE: "That day, I had surprised Maria by putting on the fur collar myself and attacking her, so to speak, when she came out of the shower. Big mistake! She was thrown, but not in the way I wanted. She sat down on the bed and glowered at me. 'I'm not a seal pup,' she said, suddenly not

playing. She took the collar and threw it under the bed. We made love that day but in the same old way, and it wasn't a happy repetition."

MARIA: "We went on for a while more or less as always, but the thing didn't turn me on any more as it had at first. The desire to start things and hunt her down just died away. I don't know why."

LEE: "I think I know why. I think you began to feel that you had been doing all the work while I could just lay back and have fun. I know I wasn't good at turning it around and initiating and so on. And you weren't good at receiving. Changing roles just didn't work for us. It was belabored. We never talked about it, maybe because there was nothing we could do, and we knew it. It wasn't in us to go back and forth from butch to femme. It was just strange that the magic of our sex play was gone, and I certainly missed it. I still do. (Turning to Maria) I still want to know what really happened to you to let that go."

MARIA: "I guess I always believed sex should be equal between women. Give and take, you know. Both give, both take. Take turns. But that never happened with Lee. She'd suddenly spring on me out of nowhere when we were both in bed reading, and well, there was no heat in it for me. She was just a clumsy bear, bungling and tickling me so that I couldn't stop laughing and she had to laugh, too. We would both be laughing so hard we'd fall off the bed! But truth be told, Lee was hurt by it. Yes, honey you were. And I was getting exasperated. I began to resent that she couldn't do it, just couldn't get it right. I mean, couldn't she learn from me, just imitate me? But no, hopeless. I guess I got hopeless about it, too. There just was no equality for us in our sex life. So I gave up on roleplay. Who needs it? We found our way around it with our big old vibrator for two. That made us perfectly equal. Top or bottom, we'd always come together and with much less work!"

LEE: "You say, top or bottom, but the funny thing is that with the toy, I enjoy being on top and Maria prefers to be the bottom. What do you make of that? She's suddenly pleased as punch to be the bottom!"

MARIA: "Maybe it's a little less exciting this way, but we are also older now and don't need so much excitement, maybe. Or rather, we prefer making it easy, which is great. We were lucky to find this way out."

LEE: "True. But I really miss our old roleplay. And now that we are getting married, this whole question is coming up again. We are different people at this point. We are beginning to understand what happened. We want to make the big commitment for the rest of our life. So why couldn't we start over and try again? Reinvent ourselves? Be the way we were?"

MARIA: (Laughing): "Reinvent ourselves and be the way we were?"

LET'S SEE...

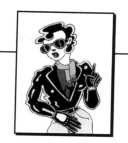

What if we tend to confuse what we mean by equality? Is it really tit for tat? I stroke your head 20 times and you nibble at my arm 20 times? Do both partners have to perform the same way and play all the same roles to feel that things are fair? When and why does difference become trouble because it is thought of as inequality?

Here was the question we asked as a group: what if Maria's disenchantment was really resentment? She didn't like this idea, but we all agreed to go after it.

Surrender for Lee seemed so easy, natural, and fulfilling. Did Maria envy Lee? Maria argued; she loved Lee so much; how could she envy her? She just wanted Lee to be able to turn it around. Why was that asking for too much? Why couldn't Lee give to her what she was able to give to Lee?

The group had another question: could Maria really be like Lee? Was Lee's gift in being turned on by anything sensual actually within Maria's reach? (Everyone got quiet. Maria got teary.)

MARIA: "You know what? That bungling bear scares the hell out of me. No way am I going to surrender to that goofy thing who can't do anything right. And I won't go on playing my Hunter role for Lee if she can't turn me into the blissed-out seal pup."

LEE: "Looks like beneath something there's always something else. So what's there for me? I mean, if I didn't bungle, I mean, if I were a powerful, irresistible hunter like Lee, how would I know when to stop? I might get really carried away and hurt you. It's scary. How could I know?"

MARIA: "Oh baby, don't tell me we're both scared?"

TOOLKIT

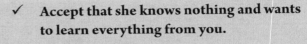

DO:

- ✓ Settle for what can be achieved.
- ✓ Appreciate what you have going for you.
- ✓ Practice if you want to learn another role.
- ✓ Practice and play, practice and play.
- ✓ Be like two kids in the sandbox.
- ✓ Be scared together. Confess.
- ✓ Make use of your toys.
- ✓ Confess your secret fantasies and fears.
- ✓ Remember, you have the best guide and teacher in bed with you.
- ✓ Admit that you know nothing and want to learn everything from her.
- ✓ Accept that she knows nothing and wants to learn everything from you.
- ✓ Find your failures funny.
- ✓ Laugh. Laughter can be an aphrodisiac.

DON'T:

- ✗ Don't mistake tit for tat for equality.
- ✗ Don't imagine you can shift roles just because you want to.
- ✗ Don't think you have to shift roles.
- ✗ Don't tell yourself you are missing out with "only" one cherished set of roles.
- ✗ Don't imagine anything new can be perfect the first time (that's Hollywood).
- ✗ Don't berate yourself for what you call your failures.
- ✗ Don't berate her for what you call her failures.

- ✗ Don't punish each other for not getting it right.

- ✗ Don't stop looking for alternatives (like your toys).

- ✗ Don't withhold sex.

- ✗ Don't forget to laugh.

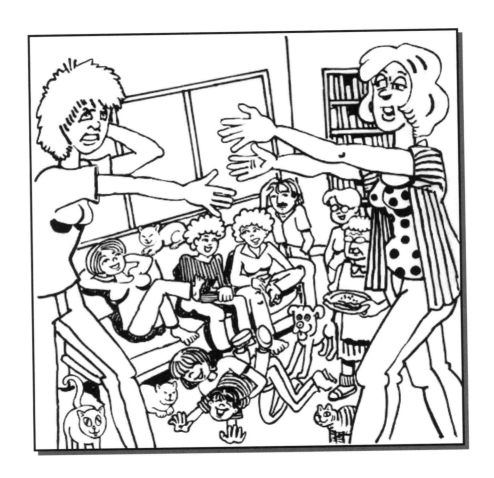

CHALLENGE 2

ONE ROOF, FOUR GENERATIONS — WOMEN WHO LOVE TOO MANY

Kim reports a story told to her in friendship.

Two mothers, each mother with two daughters. Their new family of six had been together for three years without the usual trouble of forming a blended family. The four girls had known each other from summer camp since they were kids. Both families had been through painful separations with a long period of loneliness before they got together. That was behind them, and they were a joyous household. The four girls had turned the downstairs of their new house into a single sleeping room with one bathroom and a large closet. Their friends said they always wanted to be together, and they agreed; they always wanted to be together.

The trouble began after college. They were a few years apart but were on campus at the same time and lived in the same dorm. Then, the youngest daughter fell in love with Haruko, a second-generation Japanese girl she'd met in her geology class. They decided to have a child, and after a couple of years moved back home, bringing Kenji , their little boy, with them. Over the next couple of years, one by one, the other sisters, being jealous or excluded or feeling needed by the new moms, moved back in. They all squeezed together in the downstairs space. But now instead of their old harmony there was pandemonium. The upstairs moms, who had enjoyed a couple of years more or less on their own, had been free to make love wherever and whenever. They were proud of three generations under the same roof, but was it what they wanted?

One of the mothers liked it just fine, the other didn't. She thought it was essential to go on having sex; the other thought their family commitments were more important. It did not occur to them they could ask their daughters to leave. The law of the establishment seemed to be, 'thick or thin, we stick together.'

We heard some funny stories, like the time all four sisters raced over when Kenji cried, crashing into one another in the dark. They were about to forget who the baby's actual mothers were, and they were starting to believe they could all breast-feed. Eventually, one of the other daughters brought in Ahuli, her Native American boyfriend, saying it was good for the toddler to have a father and male role model. The male role model had been raised an only child by foster-parents and liked the idea of a big "tribal" family.

It was the early nineties, a time of experimentation; they were proud of their numbers and mixed ethnicities. Their old space couldn't easily accommodate them, so they turned the closet into a small bedroom for the downstairs mothers and divided up the rest of the space by hanging lines of clothes and blankets. Our friends upstairs found they really could not make love for fear of interruption.

Things were not much better downstairs. The sisters endlessly talked about sex with Haruko and Ahuli but found that having sex with a partner felt like a betrayal of their common bond. In this free and liberal household everyone was supposed to be comfortable having sex, but no one was.

Our upstairs friends said: "Women will always give up sex if any of their relationships are threatened by it. Too bad, maybe, but that's how it is." "Well, it doesn't have to be that way, does it? Women together? Aren't we something new in the world? Why are we stuck with old rules and conditionings?" The rhetoric was good, but it fell flat. Downstairs the sisters took sides. Give up sex, not give up sex, have all the sex you want and who cares if someone overhears you?

Everyone agreed it would be better for everyone to have sex if everyone could, but some of them were certain they couldn't. Haruko came up with a schedule. Everyone would clear out of the downstairs at a fixed time, and of course they would leave their mothers time to be alone upstairs. But somehow when the prearranged time came no one was in the mood. It was artificial; it made them self-conscious; after a month, they were back to what one daughter called 'our happy nunnery.' Their older sister suggested they could become a 12 step group, 'Sexless Anonymous,' because they were obviously addicted to celibacy. Ahuli moved out. The sexless harem was just not right for the male role model.

There were other problems, but the sisters were pioneers and they persisted. Tempers flared; little Kenji was bonding exclusively with a not-mother. They talked it over and agreed the small family within their larger family would spend some time in their former closet. But no one really liked the idea, and, anyway, did it matter who Kenji believed his actual mother was? The other sisters began to show up in the closet and things went back to normal.

When the young mothers got new jobs, the others tried to put themselves on a regular care-taking plan which proved difficult for seven adults who had their own work schedules. No one thought to find a place for the little boy for a few hours in a home-care nursery. But they had to do something. The sisters were coming late to work, rushing home at lunch time, exchanging times, and forgetting the new arrangement; Kenji was a quiet child at home, but he screamed if he was taken into work with them. One of our friends upstairs, who was an immigration lawyer, was thinking about moving her office into their home. But finally, someone came up with a solution they all loved.

No one would have to move out. No one would have to give up the closet. Far from it. They would invite Omi, their mother's mother, Kenji's great-grandmother, to come live with them to take care of him. One roof, four generations. A bit crowded perhaps, but frayed tempers, celibacy and pandemonium aside, it was something to be proud of, wasn't it?

LET'S SEE...

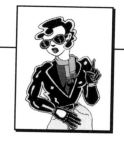

We all know similar stories. Two women have a date, the next day the proverbial U-Haul arrives carrying much more than household goods and baggage. One of the new couple's ex-lovers is sure to be not far behind, and a place will be found for her in the new establishment. Sooner or later her most recent ex will show up for an attempt at reconciliation and that's fine, too. Then the ex-lover's ex-lover, having just broken up with her lover, needs a couch for a few days, but why move on? If there are children, this whole tribe, inevitably growing bigger over time as relationships form and dissolve, will show up

for birthdays and holidays to everyone's apparent satisfaction. Is this tribal, familial bond we are so good at, taking the place of our sexuality?

Neuroscience tells us that with any sign of tension or stress women bond. Women living together, or working together in a shared space, begin to have periods (and hot flashes) at the same time. No doubt, there are women who would prefer the "happy nunnery" to any other type of living arrangement. If they are all in agreement, the "nunnery" can be happy indeed. Others would resent a situation where potentially erotic energy is dispersed over an expanding tribe of women, children, ex-lovers, and extended and blended families.

Couples often don't agree about this, but even when they do they may one day look around and ask, "Where has our sexuality gone? We've been completely eaten up, and there's nothing left for us as a couple. Where's our romance? We can't even go on vacation alone or have a date night because someone will need us or feel excluded. We never thought of ourselves as a sexless couple in a nunnery. What have we done?"

This awakening can lead to panic, claustrophobia, discord, blaming, and acting out. It can also be a wake-up call. What to do?

TOOLKIT

DO:

✓ For once, adopt the maxim that you can have it all: safety in numbers AND your couple space.

✓ Even within your couple, realize that you deserve your privacy. (You need it. You have a right to it).

✓ Protect your couple relationship as the most precious good, especially if you are parents.

✓ Consider the 50% rule of fairness: no one deserves more than half of your presence, time, or attention at any given moment (except in a crisis).

✓ Consider the Chinese formula for preserving energy: 30% for yourself, 30% for others, 30% in reserve.

✓ Work out a schedule for privacy and consider it sacred.

✓ Mediate (get the others on board) and Meditate (get yourself on board.)

✓ Get used to the idea: if you can't take care of yourself, you won't do a good job taking care of anyone else.

✓ Establish the priorities: yourself and your couple first, next the family, then others.

✓ Regularly take your lover aside to set and reset your priorities.

DON'T:

✗ Don't uphold the lame excuse that the needs of others are more important than your own.

✗ Don't sacrifice yourself: you will resent it. Resentment is the enemy of desire.

✗ Don't let anyone in your family or tribe divide you and your partner.

✗ Don't take sides against your lover and gang up on her. (If you disagree with her, do it in private.)

✗ Don't let a child or mother or ex-lover or close friend think they are more important to you than your partner.

✗ Don't tell everyone what to do and check to see if they've done it. (Micro-management: another enemy of desire.)

✗ Don't hesitate to confess as many times as possible to as many people as possible: "You know what? I just figured out I can't do everything."

✗ Don't go on believing that you or she or any of you can be perfect.

✗ Try to define what perfect means and see if you can come up with good enough.

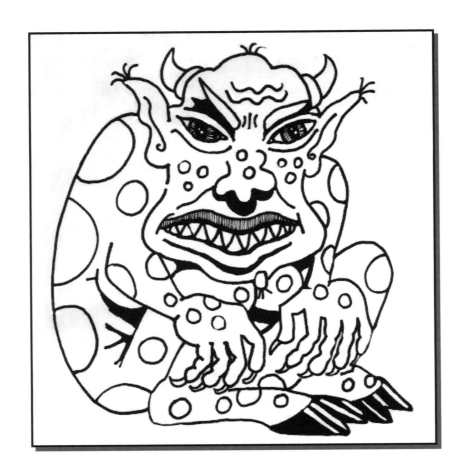

CHALLENGE 3

YOU ALWAYS, I NEVER – GRUDGES AND BED DEATH

Renate and Kim describe a session of intuitive listening.

JOELLE: I told her nothing would change if we got married. But she always has to know better. She knows everything. Hers is the only opinion that matters. She knows what kind of a dog we should get because she had that kind when she was growing up, and naturally it's the world's best type of dog. She won't believe anyone who says Cockers are inbred and can be vicious.

LAKISHA: I don't think barking at other dogs can be called vicious. That's how you exaggerate everything.

JOELLE: I heard of a Cocker Spaniel that suddenly came into the bedroom and attacked the baby.

LAKISHA: We sure don't have any baby to attack.

JOELLE: Well, we know why that is, don't we?

LAKISHA: Would you want our child being raised by a nanny like Susie and D.J.?

JOELLE: We have enough family with your folks that have to come for breakfast every Saturday.

LAKISHA: Oh honey, you know how much I love those breakfasts, and you being so sweet to my dad.

JOELLE: See? That's how she used to be when we first got together. Do you think she ever calls me honey now?

LAKISHA: I do so!

JOELLE: No, you don't. I get as much affection from you as I get from my bike pedal.

LAKISHA: She's always harping on that. Do you really think you're the same? You were so lonely and really just couldn't wait to hang with my cousins...

JOELLE: Her 16 cousins.

LAKISHA: You loved Grannie; you were always sitting next to her; you were the only one who wasn't tired of her old stories. My family welcomed you with open arms; they didn't give one thought to anyone's color.

JOELLE: Give me a break. You really think they wouldn't prefer a woman of color for you?

LAKISHA: That's not fair; it's unjust and plain lowdown. You don't have one shred of evidence. Tell me one word anyone...

JOELLE: Oh sure, words are all that count.

LAKISHA: I wouldn't mind a word or two from your folks. Do you think they might have managed a card or a telegram when we got married?

JOELLE: I told you marriage wouldn't change anything. Why should they write if they've never met you? You were so convinced that because marriage was legal now it would change their minds about us, as if legality ever overcame prejudice or racism. Honey, come on, why break your heart over this? I told you nothing would change, but you just didn't want to believe it.

LAKISHA: No, I did not. Who could believe anyone would be so pig-headed? Not to show up for their only child's wedding?

JOELLE: You could have believed it; you should have believed it. Your whole family knew what was going to happen; when did you suddenly become so naive? When we met, you knew exactly what we were getting into. You were the last person in the world to under-estimate their racism. This whole idea of marriage has turned you into something you're not and never were. Like marriage could turn your skin white and make me into god knows what you want me to be.

LAKISHA: That's insulting! Take that right back. That's your racism showing its head. You think everyone wants to turn white? If marriage did that, I would never have gotten married.

JOELLE: Well, good, then you wouldn't be so bitter and disappointed. I told you before and I told you after, marriage was not going to change me.

LAKISHA: As if anything could…

KIM REFLECTS: *Children, families of origin, parental rejection, racism, dogs, marriage with its promises and hopes. Even Snout, the Cocker Spaniel, carries the fear that their relationship could turn vicious. Joelle likes to tell a story about her family dog, a French poodle, who could pick out the best French chocolate when three or four samples were placed in front of him. This story makes Lakisha wild, but Joelle won't stop telling it. Lakisha and Joelle might have been surprised to discover that they were discussing the forbidden topic of class, until one day in the midst of their quarrel Lakisha understands. And then, all of a sudden, she understands something else.*

LAKISHA: Why do you keep harping on that ridiculous dog? Even his name could turn your stomach. Edouard, who is allowed to go into restaurants in Paris and sit on a banquette next to the family. Do you have any idea how ridiculous that sounds? I don't think anyone in my family, except maybe my cousin Lemar, could afford a plate of soup or a bone in that restaurant, but there's Edouard sitting at the table, and he probably has a bib around his neck.

JOELLE: Edouard would never need a bib. But my grandfather might.

LAKISHA: And so might you, the way you eat. Honestly, sometimes I think Granny is looking at you and wondering where you got your manners.

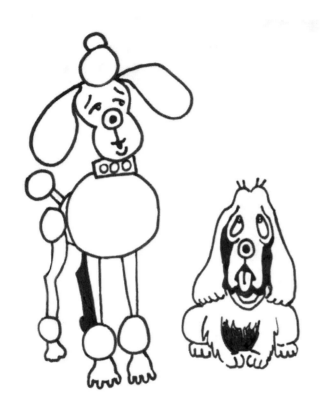

JOELLE: My manners are a rebellion, and I don't intend to change them.

LAKISHA: A rebellion? You eat like a pig because you are rebelling against your class?

There's an ominous silence, and then they both break out laughing. The idea is so absurd, and at the same time so transparently true.

LAKISHA: Edouard and Snout. I mean, just listen to their names. We've been using our dogs to hide behind. Your relatives are bluebloods from France, and I'm a darkie from Louisiana. And I'll tell you something else that's suddenly clear to me. We're furious at each other, and we can't give up a grudge because we're not all hot and on fire the way we were in the beginning.

JOELLE: Oh come on. You and your theories.

LAKISHA: You wouldn't believe how condescending you sound. What's wrong with theories? We used to sit up all night debating Freud and Jung.

JOELLE: Not that it got us anywhere.

LAKISHA: Where it got us is into a conversation which you can just damn well stop avoiding. Come on, baby.

JOELLE: Well, if all that's true... I mean, okay, we're destroying our relationship because we'd rather not have sex than have to remember what we're missing.

LAKISHA: The first time I saw you...remember you were living on that boat in Sausalito? You were playing the guitar and singing Joan Baez songs, and everyone was sitting on the floor listening, but you looked up and caught my eye...

JOELLE: It was like we were making love right there with our eyes. Everyone saw what was happening, so they just started fading away into other rooms.

LAKISHA: You could hear them laughing...

JOELLE: I didn't even have to touch you to feel the heat all over my body...

LAKISHA: Yeah... and whose fault is it that we don't have that any more?

JOELLE: If you are thinking of menopause, please think again. We could have had the same conversation long before I got my first hot flash.

LAKISHA: Sure. We always have the same conversation.

JOELLE: Okay, that's enough. You've said something new. Why fall back into the old accusations?

LET'S SEE...

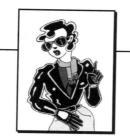

Couples come upon truths in ways that take them by surprise. "We're furious at each other, and we can't give up a grudge because we're not all hot and on fire the way we were in the beginning." "We're destroying our relationship because we'd rather not have sex than have to remember what we're missing." Could be that a whole lot of us are suffering from the same unforgiving fury hidden behind other complaints.

She never puts the cap back on the toothpaste. She uses endless amounts of toilet paper. She always drives with one foot on the brake. She will never, ever ask for directions. She gets loud and hollers about every little thing that goes wrong. She loves everyone we meet and right away invites them for dinner. She beams at all our friends but never looks at me. She always wants to make me go on vacation with her snooty parents. She spoils the dog rotten, and I always have to play the bad cop. Who has to tell our carpenters that they've messed up something? She won't. She's a god-awful cook on purpose, so I'm forced to make our meals. She always has to listen to k. d. lang when we make love. She has to have coffee first thing in the morning even if it wakes me up. She's into attachment parenting, so wouldn't you know all three kids are sleeping in our bed. She never lets me bring Sergeant Pepper, my cat, to bed.

She buys the most expensive vodka and criticizes my buying Italian goat cheese. She won't make love unless the lights are out. She's suddenly squeamish about oral sex. When I bring out our toys, she has a headache...

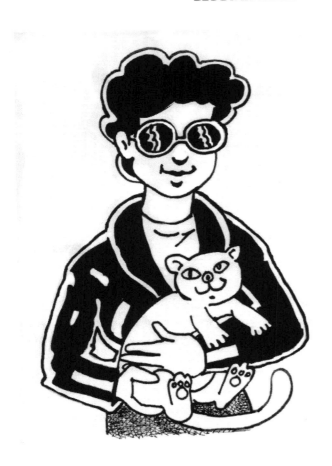

Grudges are a camouflaged expression of an inability to forgive.

When you dig a little deeper, you find a longing for closeness, intimacy, and sex, all the things that were there at the beginning and were easy and natural. Intimacy, sex, and romance have disappeared under the wear and tear of the relationship. We can't forgive each other for not being what we were in the beginning. We are deeply dismayed, puzzled, and outraged that our sexual relationship has cooled down, and we can't get it to flame up again.

Who's to blame? Obviously no one, but the grudge is standing in the way of our ability to be creative, forgiving, funny, playful, and loving. The grudge keeps us from discovering what we don't yet know about each other's and our own sexuality. Discover that and you're at the start of a new relationship.

TOOLKIT

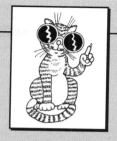

DO:

- ✓ Meet your grudges up front, get to know them well.

- ✓ Make a Grudge-List and share it with each other. (Yeah, it sounds risky but do it anyway.)

- ✓ About half way through, start to laugh.

- ✓ Recognize the patterns.

- ✓ See your grudges coming with their dramatic always-never style of speech.

- ✓ Practice saying: "Let's get out of this and be friends again."

- ✓ Put your Grudge-List on the fridge.

- ✓ Give them absurd names. ("Here comes Edouard, Snout into hiding!")

- ✓ Catch grudges at their first appearance and call them by name. ("Are we facing a manner-ism? Could we give Edouard his bib perhaps?")

- ✓ Notice how they lose their sting in the face of laughter and recognition.

- ✓ Put a dollar into a piggy bank for every time you've laughed about a grudge. (Sounds silly? But it works.)

- ✓ Go out and get something sexy with the piggy bank savings.

DON'T:

- ✘ **Don't be hard on yourself for feeling your zillion grudges.**

- ✘ **Don't feel you and she should be above such trivial pursuits.**

- ✘ **Don't expect to be further along when you need to get back to the origins of your resentments.**

- ✘ **Don't continue the tit for tat you are so good at – it does you no good.**

- ✘ **Don't agree to play the old grudge game any longer.**

- ✘ **Don't let her incite you to escalate, and don't pick up steam yourself.**

- ✘ **Don't stick around when escalation threatens.**

- ✘ **Don't get into a competition about who has fewer grudges.**

- ✘ **Don't make it a moral superiority game instead of a piggy bank frolic.**

Notes, Scribbles, Doodles

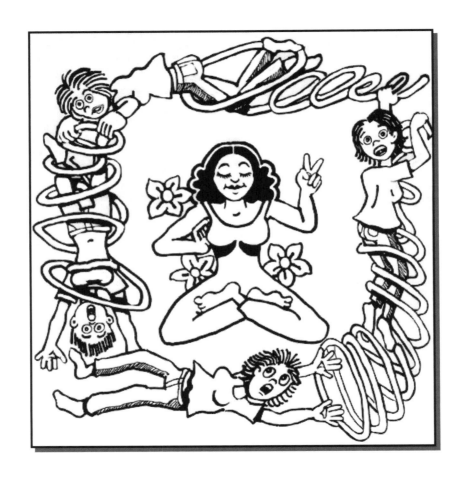

CHALLENGE 4

TIME IN, TIME OUT — THE POWER OF NEVER NOW

Part of a listening session, co-written by Kim and Renate.

Every couple we know has one continuous discussion. How do we find time for ourselves and each other? How is it possible that time goes faster and faster, and there is less and less? Is it the demands of e-mails, text messages, news on your computer, phone, Kindle, you name it? Is it the irresistible call of 350 TV channels, movies available on-demand on all your devices? The thousands of books you can sample free of charge on Amazon, or the hundreds of apps on your cell phone? The baby-can-dance YouTube jokes everyone keeps sending around? Your need to get involved in your kids' video games in order to have some even foggy idea what they are up to?

Perhaps the Age of Electronics is the Age of the End of Intimacy. And sex. Many couples with kids cannot take out even half an hour a week to talk about serious issues like expenses, parenting, or family discord. Or sex. Couples without kids? They, too, complain all the time about having no time.

Here's a couple that brings the issue to a head.

Pat never has any time, and Sean has nothing but time. Sean manages a temp agency; Pat runs a janitorial service. Both work mostly from home, and both have demands on them. Pat seems to be continually busy, driven, exasperated, and exhausted; Sean can be frequently found lying around reading, puttering in the garden, or experimenting with a new recipe. Pat is mystified by the unfairness of this difference in their daily life. When they met, Pat was cleaning houses, and Sean was a secretary, until Sean figured out that they were better at their jobs than their superiors. They could – and should -- take charge. Now Pat was irked by Sean's daylong "happy hours," and Sean was stumped by Pat's incapacity to "stop and smell the roses."

The couple described a typical day. Pat would jump out of bed and check her e-mail, worried that she might miss an opportunity in a highly competitive business. Throughout the day she kept checking her phone, texting, and showing up on Twitter and Facebook. She was able to walk out in the middle of a movie, saying it was too slow or too violent, in order not to miss anything exciting in her electronic world. There wasn't a dinner engagement without text messages coming in and being instantly returned. Wherever Pat found herself, there was a concert of beeps, buzzes, and chirps, even when she went jogging or was watching their favorite TV series in bed.

Sean would, sometimes annoyed, sometimes playfully, hide a device or turn off the volume. At other times she accused Pat of being addicted, to which Pat responded that time would tell: Sean would lose her accounts by being so "lax" and she, Pat, would have to be their sole support.

When had they last made love? Anyone's guess. Sean claimed she frequently tried to bring up the conversation; Pat thought there was no need because there was no choice. The early morning, the day, the evening, and the night were simply too short. How could she possibly dawdle in bed with Sean before everything was done?

Sean handled her business differently. In every aspect of her life, she followed a set of principles. She gave each client account a certain amount of time in the week on specified days; she was available for emergencies but otherwise didn't get involved between appointments. She had a rule that any personal correspondence had to be answered within 24 hours. There was never a pile of unfinished business in her in-box. She had learned to cut to the chase; there was no extra fat on her messages, no kind regards and warmest wishes and other niceties. She said everybody had gotten used to her style; their letters and e-mails became equally terse and could be read fast.

Speed was something Sean relished; she'd heard about "time and motion" studies when she was a student and found them fascinating. She loved to see how smoothly she could unload the dishwasher, without extra steps and movements. It went so far, Pat said, that to save time going back and forth, Sean hung up the clothes on the line with the bag of pins dangling from her neck. Her desk was neat and rather empty. Pat's was heaped with piles of paper, pens scattered everywhere, books and magazines used as markers, reminder stick-its plastering her computer, the walls, and even the front door.

If Sean lived according to the aesthetic of the minimal, Pat lived by the breathless chaos of too much. We listened to them argue about which one of them was more compulsive. Pat called Sean regimented and "anal." Sean retorted that Pat was addicted to perpetual excitement, chasing after something new even if it only was the latest email in her inbox. Sean wondered, if she was so "anal"

how did it happen that she had all this extra time to read, thumb through magazines, cook, and garden, while Pat had none?

Pat got teary. These were the things she, too, wanted and had done before they started their own business and bought a house. The way she lived now, she said, felt like an inescapable rat-race. Why hadn't Sean ever told her to do this like she did?

"Sure, like I haven't tried?" Sean replied. "Only half a million times?"

"You mean by criticizing me?"

It hadn't occurred to Sean that she could formulate a method. "My mother taught me that putting my toys and things away was like making a jigsaw puzzle; everything had a place and she made it fun to find it. I thought we were playing a game. It didn't occur to me that she was teaching me to organize."

Pat blotted her tears with a Kleenex Sean shoved over. "My house was a total pigsty. My mother couldn't even remember to pay the phone bill or the utilities. I'd come home for dinner and have to scramble for food while doing my homework and running to the neighbors to call in to the phone company. I just thought that's how things were. It's funny that I ended up cleaning people's houses. I guess I could do for them what I couldn't do as a child."

SEAN: "Oh my god, that's where your crazy multi-tasking comes from?"

PAT: "But I was always proud of it. Everyone knows that women are gifted for doing a lot of things at the same time."

SEAN: "You can't multi-task chaos. It just gets more and more chaotic. You have to start out with some order and discipline, or you'll whittle away your life. I am part of the life you're whittling away. Do you even notice that?"

PAT: "Do you ever notice how smug you sound? Maybe I want to organize things, too. But I don't know where to start, and you are not helping me."

Now they both look helpless. What can they do?

LET'S SEE...

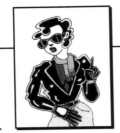

This is the record of a single, two-hour talk, unusual for the speed in which the crucial issues arose and were engaged. Who would have imagined that Sean had been taught as a child to live by a definite set of principles? Or that Pat's chaos was depriving her of erotic and many other pleasurable experiences? Chaos and spontaneity had always sounded sexy to Pat. She feared to be caged in by order and become "anal." She could hardly believe that her disorder was robbing her of a sensual life.

Sean hadn't noticed how proud she was of her own disciplined way of going about things. It seemed natural to her, but it also set her apart from "most other people" who could never, she said, "get on top of their life." Most other people? Or, was it Pat she had in mind?

Would it have occurred to her sooner to teach Pat her method if she hadn't taken a secret pleasure in Pat not knowing how to straighten out her desk? We didn't ask this question; it was asked by Sean. She recognized that "a couple isn't always the couple's best teacher." Sometimes outside support has to be called on. Sean and Pat began to try on practical ideas. A professional organizer might have to come in to sort things out, starting with Pat's desk. There would still be room for Sean to help Pat keep a schedule, but first Sean would have to sweep the condescension out of her critical advice. Pat would have to re-experience thrills and excitements different from rushing after the next tweet. She would have to try out a certain amount of tight-laced discipline in order to find time for relaxation and pleasure. Time for sex.

PAT: "Schedule sex? You think that's sexy? I think the three of you might really be off your rockers."

SEAN: "You don't schedule sex; you schedule time for fun."

And what would fun mean? Unplug and "smell the roses"? Enjoy the sunset with a drink? Parallel play, reading a gardening article together, watching a cooking show without interruption?

Pat resisted. "All that sounds forced. Like being force-fed."

"Come on honey," Sean insisted, "if I interrupted your computer binging by bringing in your Three Sisters caramel fudge ice cream, be honest, you'd love it."

PAT: "But you never do. When have you ever done that? You just lay around reading magazines and feeling superior."

SEAN: "Okay, I'll put it on my schedule. Ten minutes for bringing Three Sisters caramel fudge on a tray. Ten minutes to enjoy it together."

PAT: "Eight, because you'll need two to clear it away."

SEAN: "Okay, we'll add in five minutes to smooch a bit."

Finally, laughter. And a new possibility. Was Pat about to discover that what had seemed "anal" could turn out to be erotic? Maybe, we thought, you really could schedule in spontaneity.

What's the moral of this story? Time is like freedom; no one gives it to you, you have to take it.

TOOLKIT

DO:

- ✓ Stop.

- ✓ Intimacy, sex, work, family, friends, playtime: you can have it all if you time yourself.

- ✓ Figure out how much sex and intimacy you both want.

- ✓ Fantasize about the erotic potential of making time.

- ✓ Remember: the time for spontaneity can be scheduled (just like you schedule a weekend away).

- ✓ Unplug all electronic devices.

- ✓ Enjoy being unreachable.

- ✓ Reap the rewards of cultivating time.

- ✓ Keep to an online diet.

- ✓ Add up your electronic calories (how many do you really need?)

- ✓ Go cold turkey on just one soap opera or cooking show; sit out just one sports series.

- ✓ Be ruthless with your priorities.

- ✓ Sit down and meditate the minute you have no time.

DON'T:

- ✗ Stick to the Do's, and the Don'ts won't matter.

Notes, Scribbles, Doodles

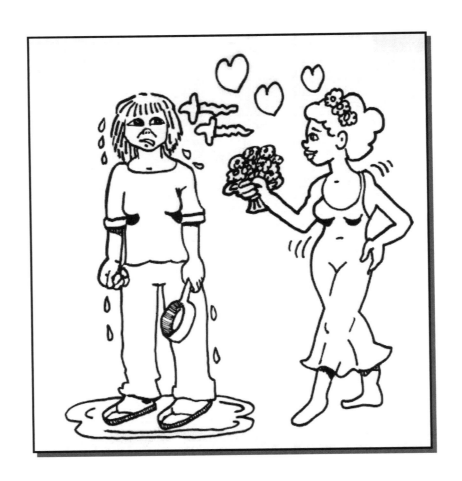

CHALLENGE 5

THE RAVENOUS BEAST — SEX AFTER MENOPAUSE?

A condensation of a heated monologue from a listening session, reconstructed by Kim and Renate.

ANIKA: What to do? Hormone replacement for menopause was suddenly not advisable any more. All my friends went off, so okay, I'll try it. Time-warp back four years: violent hot flashes once again, night sweats, monster moods, biting the heads off everyone at the slightest provocation. "Mom, what's for dinner tonight?" "We'll find out when you make it." Was that me? No. I didn't recognize myself and no one around me recognized me either.

Maybe it was the reappearance of my mother? When I and my girl friends were trying out our first bras and Kotex, our mothers were turning into furies, banging and clanging the pots and pans in the kitchen, constantly nagging, barely containing their bad moods with furious scrubbing. Was I becoming like my mother? No way. I ran to my

doctor. Help me, save me. I'm being taken over by my Dutch mother.

"Well, apart from replacement hormones, we have good experience with anti-depressants," my doctor says. "You'd take the minimal dose. Only 5% of people have side effects." Side effects? I was immediately suspicious. What side effects? "It can happen that it slows orgasm. But it's really rare."

I'd never gone near antidepressants. In my Dutch culture you just tough it out. But now that we'd been in the new world for several generations, I mean, why not? I said to myself, it's just an experiment. If it doesn't work, you go off again. Right? No harm done. I was curious about it. What if the side-effects for me would be a better mood? Ha ha! My hot flashes were gone over night even before the medication was supposed to kick in.

Unfortunately, something else was gone, too, over night. It was as if someone had drawn a curtain across the sex-zone of my brain. I had almost no desire left. Orgasm became a long-distance runner. It was a torture, always just about to occur, fading back, building up again, an endless hovering. My sweetheart and I had been great at developing the technique of a quickie for sexual release. The busier we got with kids and jobs and all, the faster we would reach for our toys. Instant nirvana. Our motto was, "Get to the goal the easy way." But what if there was no goal any more?

I had plunged right in to the 5%. Why me? My mother's curse? I was sure of it. Here I was falling back into my miserable twenties when sex meant always lagging behind my quick-to-come lovers. Feeling inadequate, second-rate, getting more self-conscious by the minute. What if my sinking sexual self-esteem was more of a damper than the drug? Would I once again be tempted to fake it?

My lover, who had no problem coming said, "Oh, don't worry. Sex isn't that important after all. Just think how much of it we've already had over the years." That comforted me for a moment but didn't convince me. I could just as well say, "Well, at our age, life isn't all that important either. Just think how much of it we've already had over the years." "Oh," she said, giving me a look. "Sex is essential for life?" It was.

For me, sex is much more than sex. I began to lecture the minute we got into bed. "You can't be serious, letting us give up sex. I'm telling you, without sex there's no real intimacy for me. Tenderness alone doesn't do it. You know it yourself. Sex, now that's a risk. You never know the outcome. Desire and surrender, that's what I love about it, doing something daring. But you know me. Love for me can be so intense I don't know what to do with myself. I'm overwhelmed with lust, enthusiasm, greed, the whole nine yards. Sometimes I feel like I want to take your body and knead it like dough, tear it into pieces, bite whole chunks out of it. I mean, possess and swallow you whole in order to – I don't know. Finally be satiated? What would I do with these feelings without sex?"

She was definitely listening. "How about starting a fight?"

"Exactly. When you come right down to it, desire is a beast, a ravenous beast. If we don't feed it, we can be sure it's gonna turn against us."

I got off the Effexor, declaring that I'd rather have hot flashes than give up on sex. If the bad moods would return, let them. I'd been too much of a good-girl all my life anyway. I would endure any discomfort, even clanging and banging in the kitchen, rather than renounce what to me was the meaning of life. My sweetie went along with me. She never minded when I was in a bad mood. She liked a bit of edginess in me. She convinced our kids to join in. "She's at it again. Watch out for the flying pan."

We made a pact. We would have twice as much sex as usual to make up for any clanging symptoms I would come up with. We discovered ice. The little cubes that play hot and cold on a flushed body. And guess what, my moods improved. So what if I was sweaty and had a few bad nights a week! Sex was worth it.

We encouraged our kids to accept invitations to sleep-overs, and we took off for Boston. We invented a game. A chance meeting in some cheap hotel. We'd dress up, take separate tables in the dining room. We'd notice each other, begin to secretly observe, move on to inviting glances, send over a glass of champagne. The waiters played along. A little note, the plastic flower from our table, a napkin with a lipstick trace dropped surreptitiously on the way to the ladies' room. One of us (we never knew which) joined the other at her table. The one who arrived had to play a game of seduction against a game of resistance until finally she could slip her key across the table. And leave.

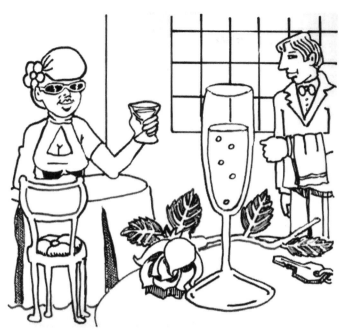

We liked our game so much that we didn't give it up when my hot flashes died down, and I went back to being a recognizable people-pleaser. By then I was so good at dressing up and using disguise. There was this one time when I swear she didn't recognize me and was embarrassed by this strange woman flirting with her. Not that she'll ever admit it. In Massachusetts, gay marriage had been legal for years, and we couldn't make up our minds. But once we discovered how to re-invent our sex life, we weren't afraid to get hitched (as our teenage son loved to call it). We rounded up the kids, got dressed up, and took off for City Hall.

LET'S SEE...

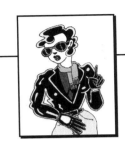

Maybe we give up too easily. What if no one ever told us sex would dry up after menopause? Suppose we believed that a woman's sexuality gets stronger as she ages? Never mind hormones and physiology, we are not our chemistry. After all, sexual excitement and release can be achieved simply by thinking and imagining. The ability to fantasize does not end with menopause.

Forget dryness, there's always sexy lubricant; forget sagging bodies, bodies always look great in the horizontal. If you're especially self-conscious, who says you have to get undressed? Would you really give up sex because you're afraid to let her know you'd rather keep your clothes on?

We are told: now that you're getting old, you are not desirable. If you can't be desired, you won't be able to desire. The cultural message is: "It's all over Baby, better accept it."

What an idea. Enough to bring on hot flashes.

This unholy message shows up when many women have finally reached empowerment. We are getting on in our careers, are done with child-rearing, for the first time perhaps we are focused on our selves. And now, right now, we're told it's all over? It's equally hard to believe and not believe this absurdity. Empowerment always extends beyond cultural norms and into the body. Desire, even if less urgent, has to be known as what it is now. Who says that pleasure comes to an end at the age of forty-five? Maybe hot flashes would feel a lot different if they didn't mean the alleged end of passion.

TOOLKIT

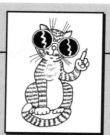

DO:

- ✓ Rebel.

- ✓ Claim.

- ✓ Insist.

- ✓ Pursue.

- ✓ Invent.

- ✓ Get a little obsessed.

- ✓ Get a lot obsessed.

- ✓ Cultivate fantasies.

- ✓ Play games.

- ✓ Get your partner involved (try all of the above).

- ✓ Re-claim your youthful lust (alone and together).

- ✓ Cherish your changing body. (Who knows what it will become?)

- ✓ Take heart from the ancient images of big-bodied women. Notice their tired breasts, big bellies, and big thighs (all meant to be worshiped).

- ✓ Regenerate.

- ✓ Remember: you can be a born-again sexual woman.

DON'T:

×   Don't believe anything you've been told about women.

×   Don't believe anything you've been told about aging.

×   Don't believe anything you've been told about sex.

×   Don't think you are defined by your hormones.

×   Don't give up; don't give in.

×   Don't act out with anyone half your age (it gets tired fast).

×   Don't berate yourself if your sex drive changes (everything changes).

×   Don't berate your lover.

×   Don't accept "bed-death" without fighting back.

Notes, Scribbles, Doodles

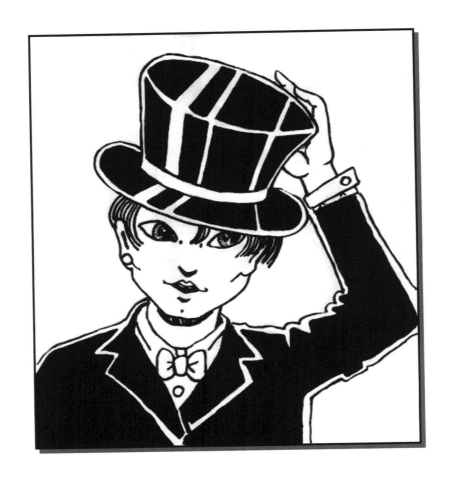

CHALLENGE 6

MYTHS OF DESIRE – PASSION AND PAIN VS. PLEASURE

Renate's story followed by a dialogue with Kim.

As a young lesbian I felt I had to turn into a "boy." I was thin and athletic. In a jeans outfit, my hair cut very short, I looked like a boy and set out to court women without getting "involved." In Paris, where I lived, the height of the erotic feminist wave was attracting countless women--all kinds of women, not just lesbians. Faster than anyone could think, everyone was turned on by everyone. The era of couples seemed over.

Looking back, all of us were experimenting with freedom: freedom to desire, freedom of choice, freedom from "relationship coffins" and gender roles. The myth of passion in our culture is about longing for the unreachable or forbidden lover (think of *Anna Karenina* or *Gone with the Wind*). Passion is about the mysterious stranger, pining for sexual fulfillment that is seductively offered but remains elusive, there for a moment, then out of reach.

I chose lovers who were available one night and distant the next, allowing me to be in a constant state of arousal, pursuing them. I had never been more turned on or felt more empowered than in this active, "boyish" affirmation of my sexual desire. If a woman pursued me in turn, I tried to convince her to cultivate a distance, a degree of withholding, to make sure our desire would drive us wild. I kept looking for lovers who would be able, at the height of our sexual affair, to withdraw and force me to wait and pine.

These amorous pursuits against real and artificial obstacles seemed to me the essence of passion. Passion has to come with pain, we are taught, and sex is hottest when painful longing is released for a brief moment of ravishment -- a one night stand, a conquest without consequence, an adventure for adventure's sake.

I was traveling for a time, presenting a radical lesbian multimedia show that I had written and created with my last long-term lover. I was sailing across Europe from one women's festival and women's center to another. My Parisian friends were joking that I had "a woman in every port." It took me a few years to realize how exhausting this passion-play was, how little satisfaction it brought in the end to everyone involved.

I finally began to wonder if sexual conquest for its own sake was as predictable and repetitive as sex in a steady relationship. I also had to admit that I didn't manage all that well to keep my distance when I was turned on by a lover. When sex is good, really good, one wants it again, and then again. One naturally gets attached to the person who is so hot. One is tempted, falls in love, and promptly slides into the new relationship. But hot sex doesn't mean one is otherwise compatible, likes the other's opinions, politics, lifestyle, friends, etc.

Disappointments and heartaches were the unavoidable outcome of my trying to "love like a boy," but I knew nothing better. I had an inkling about the deeper failures of my quest: my innate yearning for love and romance remained unfulfilled. My heart remained lonely. I didn't believe I would ever meet the woman with whom love and sex could be different, inspiring, never boring-- in short, the soul-mate.

So I went on in my not so merry ways -- until I met Kim. She, it turned out, had an idea. It wasn't anything she had experienced, and she had never told it to anyone. She said there had to be an altogether different kind of passion, one that was not linked to the pain of tormented pining. It had to do with pleasure, pure sensual body pleasure, revealed in the most intimate, honest confessions of a long-term relationship. Kim put a question to both of us. Why shouldn't sex between two women who are radically honest remain the hottest sex known to women?

LET'S SEE...

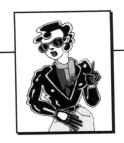

RENATE: "If that were possible, all the shame, guilt, fear, inhibition that's in the way of pleasure would have to be peeled away, layer by layer. That's a tall order. How would you do that?"

KIM: "We would have to figure it out together. But one thing I suspect: if you could go beyond this shame and inhibition you would come to a sensuality so fierce and tender you most likely wouldn't have felt it since you were a little kid."

RENATE: "You probably aren't talking about a regression to something infantile. It sounds like a retrieval or rescue of a capacity that's been left behind in our growing up."

I remembered that one of the greatest sensations of bliss in my early childhood was sitting at my mother's knees while she was talking to someone with her fingers absent-mindedly stroking my hair. There was such wonder in this touch that the memory stayed with me, deep in my body. Of course, as I grew older, my mother wouldn't think of stroking my hair while I was at her knees with company present. Or on any other occasion. Childhood bliss was done with. No lover I've met as an adult ever brought this sensation back to me. I was unable to teach or even reveal this embarrassing "childish" desire. Telling my lover would have taken away the magic of its happening out of nowhere, out of the blue, as it did in childhood.

KIM: "I remember something similar. Before my sister died, when I was four and a half years old, she used to hold me on her lap while she was typing and nibble at my ears. When she died, I couldn't bear to even think of this. I certainly wouldn't think of asking a grownup lover to enact this tender sensuality. I mean, ask her to let me sit on her lap while she is at her computer and command her to nibble?"

RENATE: "Exactly. This is what we do to our most intense body pleasures. Most of them are from childhood and we assume they can never be brought into the present. We find them absurd, make fun of them, belittle them, tell ourselves to get over them. Grow up already."

KIM: "Well, okay. I guess we assume we have to forget our original body with its extraordinary capacity for pleasure."

RENATE: "Maybe it's never forgotten, just... I don't know. Buried? Hidden away in some forbidden cave? The question is: how to recover this lost capacity for pleasure? Wouldn't it mean uncovering all the most intimate secrets our bodies are keeping -- sometimes even from ourselves?"

KIM: "Hell, yes. It could go on for a whole lifetime, a whole marriage, without ever getting repetitive! I bet there'll always be another sensual secret the body has been holding back, some corner for what seems an illicit desire, hungry to be known."

RENATE: "Do you think it has ever been done?"

KIM: "Who knows. You want to try?"

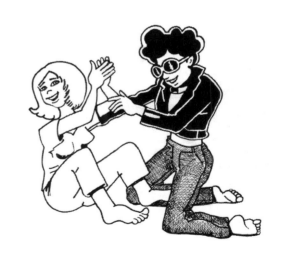

TOOLKIT

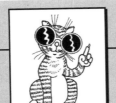

DO:

- ✓ Redefine pleasure.

- ✓ Question the old adage: "Without pain, no pleasure!"

- ✓ Question the pain that masquerades as desire.

- ✓ Go straight for pleasure and fulfillment.

- ✓ Remember rolling around in wild sensations when you were a kid.

- ✓ Bring your shames and inhibitions to your lover.

- ✓ Be confessional. Be confessional.

- ✓ Find a time to whisper secrets (your body has so many).

- ✓ Tell fears and longings never told before.

- ✓ If you don't feel your desire is hot enough, tell a risqué truth (go ahead, try it).

DON'T:

- ✕ Don't take your longings outside the relationship (unless both of you agree to do so. But then:)

- ✕ Don't underestimate your capacity for jealousy.

- ✕ Don't think that painful desire is the hottest desire on earth.

- ✕ Don't let Hollywood passion-myths distract you (unless you and your lover like to play them out).

✗　Don't believe that "real" passion is a dead-serious matter.

✗　Don't believe that infantile moods, giggles, laughter, aren't part of hot sex.

✗　Don't forget to bring your childhood fantasies into your couple play.

✗　Don't think that cuddling can't lead directly into sex.

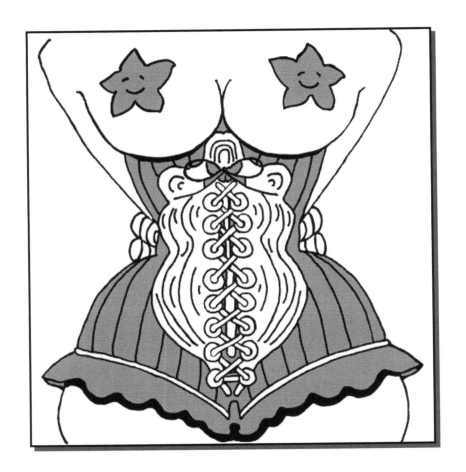

CHALLENGE 7

THE GENITAL CORSET – LOOSEN UP

Co-written by Kim and Renate directly after a couple's session.

A couple came to see us. On the phone they made it clear they wanted to work with both of us. They were so opposed, they said, it would be impossible for one person to do them both justice.

To our surprise they walked in hand in hand. Andi, tall, athletic, with a bold and striking face. Grace, a head smaller, with a soft body and an apologetic smile on her round face. Andi says, "So which of you is on my side?" They laugh and exchange a kiss. "Pick one," Renate says and Grace scurries over to sit near Kim. "I'm so glad you look like you do, I was afraid you'd be a toughy." "Okay," Andi says with an exaggerated sigh, "I guess I'm stuck with Renate." They look at Renate to make sure the joke has worked. It has and Andi begins talking.

ANDI: "We just had our twentieth anniversary. And I thought, by god, twenty years. This is enough; I should be allowed to make a move. For her sake, I mean. After twenty years wouldn't it be time for an orgasm?"

(Grace inches closer to Kim)

ANDI: "I'm always the one; I initiate; I make love to her, and I know I'm a darned good lover. She's not the first woman I've been with. I know what to do, but no result. She won't come, she just won't. I don't have to tell you the million things I've tried. Let's just cut to the chase."

KIM: "Is the only permissible result an orgasm?"

Both look shocked.

ANDI: "Well, it's natural, it's healthy, I mean, how could you not? Something must have happened in her childhood." (We glance at Grace, but she isn't saying a word.) "I mean, all our friends suggested the same thing, so finally I gave in and went to Good Vibrations. We have a local store. And then for our anniversary I brought her breakfast to bed, a tray, coffee, red roses and that big, brown bag with a pink heart I had taped to it." Andi shakes her head. "She opens it, looks in the box and doesn't know what it is. No, I mean it, she doesn't know what it is. So, she says, 'O boy, I'm getting a massage for our anniversary.'" (Grace has shrunk into her seat. Andi frowns at her). "So, cut to the chase, it did nothing for us. I'm the only one who plays with it."

Grace, with a winning smile, glances at Kim, "But I tried, didn't I?"

ANDI: "She did; she tried; I'll give her that. But I give up. There's really something wrong with her. Something must have happened in her childhood. I'm absolutely sure it did." She gets up suddenly and kneels down next to Grace. "Baby, you look hurt. I never want to hurt you, you know that."

GRACE: "I've had it, too. You always have to make me. It's never good enough for you; twenty years of bugging me and then this vibrator thing. You never even notice that I'm perfectly happy.

I miss nothing. But you just won't believe it. So maybe, yes, something happened and maybe it did not. But one thing is for sure, it's not defining the rest of my life. That's what you're doing."

RENATE: "Let's see if we've understood." (Turning to Andi) "You think Grace's orgasm is crucially missing from your relationship. Grace says that she's perfectly happy, and you don't believe her. We understand, Andi, that you want to make Grace even happier than happy. Grace, is there anything Andi could give you that would make you happier than happy?"

GRACE: (Looking at Andi, tears in her eyes) "There is, honey. In our early days, a couple of times you gave me a foot massage. I didn't even have to ask. It was such bliss I thought I'd die."

KIM: "You never told her?"

ANDI (bursting in): "A foot massage? You call that sex? Bliss? Is that an orgasm? I mean, okay, if you could manage to come from baby stuff like that, well, okay, fine with me. But would you? Of course not."

RENATE: "Do you feel that Grace is deliberately holding something back from you? Trying to deprive you?"

Andi frowns, uncertain how to answer.

GRACE (startled): "But I would never. Why would I? I always want to give you everything I have."

KIM: "But you don't have an orgasm to give?"

This strikes all of us as very funny. Andi and Grace obviously enjoy laughing together.

RENATE: "What's so terrible about never having an orgasm? It sounds like you have everything else."

GRACE: "No. I don't have a foot massage. But do I hold that against her?"

ANDI (looking stricken): "But you never told me you wanted a foot massage."

GRACE: "Oh, I've told you a hundred million times, but you don't take it in because you have to always go you know where and try to make me."

ANDI: "Okay then, are you saying I should take this vibrator and give her a foot massage?"
The tone of sheer uncomprehending puzzlement makes us all laugh. But that is what we seem to be saying.

LET'S SEE...

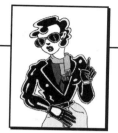

RENATE: We are locked into the belief that sex and sexual fulfillment have to be genital. But we know that is a false belief and maybe more true to a man's experience.

We know of women who can come simply by thinking or fantasizing their way to an orgasm, and others who are in ecstasy in their bodies without any kind of orgasmic release. What do we make of that? Why do we all squeeze ourselves into this "genital corset?" The whole rest of the body is fenced out for maximum, genital predominance. Here reigns the genital queen detached from her people! You know all those other places of desire that are not supposed to be "erogenous zones"-- like the neck, ears, knees, underarms, elbows, feet, you name it.

KIM: Sometimes I think there are two profoundly distinct types of sexual experience. Freud thought the normal and desirable development was to progress from what he called the polymorphous perversity of children to genital predominance. By "polymorphously perverse" he meant the child's capacity to take pleasure all over the body before genital experience became predominant. Really? Perverse? Maybe he was describing male sexuality, and maybe not even that.

But for women, as we know if we're paying attention, sexual desire remains distributed throughout an "equal-opportunities" body. You know what I mean? No one part legislated as superior to another in terms of pleasure. And I don't care how many nerve endings the clitoris has when compared with the foot. Is it nerve endings alone that determine pleasure?

RENATE: That's what I'm getting at. Extreme pleasure in the body has an orgasmic quality to it, which we tend to ignore because it doesn't fit into the genital queen's corset. This is another cultural gap, a real failure to take in how women are made.

KIM: We've been yammering on and on for decades about the discovery of what it means to be a woman. Well, by god here's another one of those discoveries. Grace is really introducing a radical and perhaps new idea, that sexual fulfillment can mean blissful touch no matter where it takes place. Who the hell gets to define what is sexual and what is not? Is that what you mean by the "genital corset"?

RENATE: If Grace's feet were touched in the right way, couldn't it be a turn-on for both of them? What would stop Andi from coming as she's giving Grace such pleasure? It might never have occurred to her.

KIM: There's something about touch. A friend of mine talks about "skin hunger," the longing of the skin for touch. She misses it more than anything else when she's not with a partner. The skin is an erogenous zone and not given enough credit. It craves, it desires, it longs for contact and stimulation, it has its preferred places, its ecstasy of fulfillment when enough is enough and its longing is satisfied. Who is to say this isn't orgasmic? I mean, an increasing intensity of sensual desire, which reaches a peak of satisfaction and then drops down. Not only men, women, too, tend to rush past the sensual-body to the genitals. Aren't we missing something?

RENATE: Foreplay? But there's something wrong with that notion. Foreplay suggests touching, stroking, smooching come before the essential play, like the mere appetizer before the main dish. Foreplay could be a supreme play in which the entire body is invited to participate. The crucial thing is pleasure, isn't it?

KIM: What are we getting at? Are we saying sex doesn't survive in our lesbian relationships because we're thinking about it in too narrow a way? That we don't cultivate a woman's capacity for so-called polymorphous pleasure–which is certainly not perverse and definitely not left behind in childhood?

RENATE: We're always going back to childhood.

KIM: Of course, nothing is lost or left back there if we approach it the right way. Re-inventing pleasure may take inventiveness, unconventional thinking, an appetite for play.

RENATE: Maybe we can get away from, "good god, how long it takes her!" Don't we hear that complaint all the time? Sex becomes laborious, desire flees, bed-death is looming. But if there's no pre-set, tyrannical, genital goal, what could take too long? Taking pleasure?

KIM: And look what we would get. Sexual desire that has freed itself from the corset. The discovery of what we really want instead of what we're taught we ought to want. Good gracious, we're talking about life-long, intensely compelling, sexy marriages between women. If there are couples who don't believe this, I dare them to go and try it. The proof, as we all know, is in the pudding.

TOOLKIT

DO:

✓ Make sure you know what you want and desire. (If you don't know, figure it out.)

✓ Every woman is made in her unique way; lovers have to discover what that is.

✓ Redefine for yourself (yourselves) what sex is and what is sexy to you.

✓ Recognize skin-hunger. Indulge it.

✓ Rediscover your equal-opportunities body.

✓ Call it "all lustful pleasures welcome all over the skin."

✓ Break out of the genital corset at least from time to time.

✓ Discover the orgasmic potential of simple touch anywhere the body craves it.

✓ Play together without ulterior motives.

✓ Ramp up the cuddle if you are cuddle bears.

✓ When your friends brag about their orgasms, exchange a knowing smile.

✓ Think again if you think anyone is taking too long. Grab that vibrator.

DON'T:

✗ Don't buy into the cultural notion that genital sex is the only real sex.

✗ Don't judge the absence of orgasm as failure.

✗ Don't chase unicorns: the perfect, instantaneous, all-fulfilling, "Technicolor" Orgasm.

✗ Don't forget pleasure is everywhere at hand.

✗ Don't go on and on if either one of you seems to be taking too long. (Don't leave that vibrator in the back of the drawer.)

✗ Don't enter the competitive race to orgasm.

✗ Don't think you aren't missing something (you are) even if you're a celebrated orgasmic speed train.

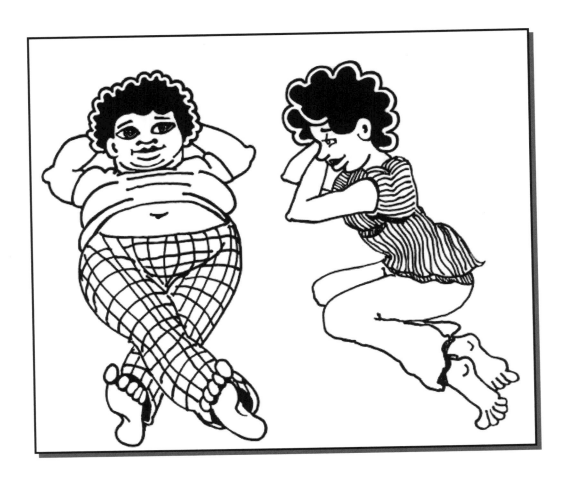

CHALLENGE 8

THE OTHER WOMAN — HOT BURN/SLOW BURN

Kim's confession.

When Renate and I had been together for thirteen years, we faced a crisis. Actually, I was the crisis and in a crisis; our relationship felt the stress of it and might have ended. We called the crisis Falling in Love with a Younger Woman. My friends who heard about it thought I was mad. I agreed. Renate's friends who heard about it thought she was crazy to be so understanding. With that we both did not agree.

In our 13 years together, we had followed a consistent principle. We told the truth. So that's what we did now. We avoided lies, secrecy, and evasions. Renate was heart-broken but determined to figure out what was going on. Why in the world was her beloved soul-mate behaving in a way that was so out of character?

We both remembered our four-hour phone calls from Berkeley to Paris. I, after all, had been the champion of monogamy. There was a mystery here, and we both had to understand it. Day by day we communicated our feelings—Renate's sense of being in an earthquake, not knowing where to turn, where to go, what to do if we separated. She had given up her life in Europe to be with me. How could this be happening if we were meant to be together forever?

Renate came to the conclusion that whatever I was doing, it could have nothing to do with our relationship. It was my own private madness, and she would do her best to see me through it. But slowly, she began to prepare to take on life alone again. During the year and a half I was caught up with The Younger Woman, we were careful to preserve whatever we could of our relationship. We got a place for Renate in the same neighborhood within walking distance. We met several times a week to take our usual night walk in the Berkeley hills. We still went to the opera and ballet together.

So what was I doing? I had fallen into an obsession with a woman I had met at a friend's book party. I didn't understand it at the time. I couldn't describe it. She was a dark-haired woman with an exotic, beautiful face, dark-skinned in the way some Jewish women are, with dark, dreamy eyes. Her face expressed a faint hope that this stranger she was speaking with might change her life. I had lost an older sister as a child who looked a great deal like this woman. I had always cherished a secret conviction she would come back to me. Was this the way she would return? So much younger than I was because during the years she was dead I had gone on living?

For The Younger Woman the fantasy was different. It transposed us into high-school sweethearts. The entire year and a half we were together we lived these fantasies. Sometimes she was my sister for whom I had waited those fifty years; sometimes I was an adolescent boy head over heels in love with my first girlfriend, who would gaze at me with her searching, troubled eyes that promised to fulfill all desires if only I would rescue her. In reality she was thirty-eight, a year younger than my daughter. In our fantasy she was still living with a violent father and longing for a mother who had disappeared.

Our entire sexual relationship was spun from fantasies of return and rescue, separation, loss, and rediscovery. I'm not sure there was a single encounter in which we were ourselves of the present: she a mother of a young child; I in my fifties and wholeheartedly involved with my life-companion and soul-mate.

The sexual intensity of an adolescent boy is a serious matter. I had never experienced it before. Yet now, in the way these things are possible when they disregard time, I had slipped free of my many years. When we were apart we couldn't wait to get back together; we wrote e-mails and left messages and made plans to meet. When I was with Renate, I never thought of her. I was unable to think of her;

I could scarcely remember her. Renate and I were reality; The Younger Woman and I belonged to a make-believe erotic world.

We know that these things, whatever they are, can't go on forever; they all begin in the same way, in the unfolding of a story we are telling ourselves while we are living it. But the endings have their unique torque and are often unexpected. I was brought out of my enchantment by memory of Renate. It seemed strange at first that the sensual quality of our thirteen years had managed to rise up against the heady power of adolescent yearning. For a time, the two seemed to run neck and neck, but gradually memory began to win out.

My body remembered itself in Renate's touch as the body of a mature woman. My hands began to recall the shape of Renate's shoulders. I remembered the way her long legs wrapped around me; I missed her feet with their serious toes we had called pilgrims for the way they seemed about to start out on a long journey. The relationship with The Younger Woman ended of its own accord, fading back into the fantasy from which it had emerged. She got involved with someone else as I went back to Renate.

Once back together, Renate said she bore no grudge because everything had been honestly spoken between us. She thought it possible the ghost of the dead sister had finally been put to rest. I was eager to express an awareness of the pain my relationship with this dark-eyed phantom had caused. We both agreed I had done everything I could to exorcise the obsession. Nevertheless, she felt shaken.

She kept an inner reserve and caution until she was convinced that our relationship could once again be trusted. "Can you really come back to what we have after a hot, new sexual relationship with a younger woman?" She'd dared to ask, not sure how I would answer. Even I was not sure and then in the next instant I was. Yes, I could come back. Both of us present, vulnerable in truth and in reality. The depth of love and recognition in body and spirit. The sure knowledge of where and when to touch and how much and how little. This touch that conveyed the fierce and tender history of our thirteen years together.

LET'S SEE...

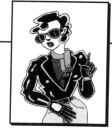

In our crisis, what had looked like a major betrayal wasn't what it seemed. We had to remind ourselves that a couple is made of two individuals, each with her own path in life. And that each path can encounter snags and obstacles that will, of course, greatly affect both partners. Remaining with our lover or returning to her after an affair is a sexual challenge. The wild, hot energies of the affair can make the slower burn of our long-term sexuality seem comparatively dull. But is that "safe but boring" sex really all there is?

We started to think about the Hot Burn versus the Slow Burn.

The Hot Burn is the quick flare, the instantaneous sexual kindle, the experience we think worth ruining our lives for. The Slow Burn takes longer to get going. It needs a more intimate, mature knowledge of our lover's body. It requires patience as the heat gathers and gains force. The great temptation of the Hot Burn is that you race ahead of yourself and seem transformed. Your old self is left behind. You are carried beyond the sexual limitations that have always plagued you. How could you resist it?

The Slow Burn is mostly ignored because it is compared to the Hot Burn and found wanting; we don't cherish it because we almost don't notice it. After the Hot Burn you return to yourself. You come back to the person you have always been in all your sexual shyness, shame, and fear. Back to your serious doubt of your attractiveness. Your body's repressions and secrets speak up again. The Slow Burn never really gets a chance; before it can develop, we have to face everything the Hot Burn has allowed us to leave behind. Poor old Slow

Burn, personally and culturally unrecognized as a possibility of sexual fulfillment.

Renate said, you can be sure Tristan and Isolde, who had been drugged into their passion, knew nothing about it. I said, ditto for Romeo and Juliet, those kids of thirteen and sixteen with their single burning night together. Renate said, Anthony and Cleopatra; I said, Paris and Helen of Troy; she said, Eloise and Abelard. You didn't even have to know their stories to know how hot they'd been burning. Did two women together have to be walled in by these old bedtime stories?

Let's think: what would have happened to Romeo and Juliet ten years later if they had lived, and lived together? Romeo might be taking off for Padua every chance he got, resenting the time Juliet spent with their children; she might have felt that after a day of kids and the house and her own family another demand on her for intimacy was just too much. Could she have taught Romeo to caress her tired body to sleep? To give her a sexy foot massage that would have melted her to the bone?

Lesbian sex manuals are filled with suggestions for lovers to get back into the Hot Burn: fill the bubble bath, light the candle, burn your incense, get out that exotic oil, slide your k. d. lang into the CD player. Start with the back rub.

All this sudsing would be well and good if the attempt to reach a Hot Burn weren't so misguided. Candles light up the Slow Burn. Think of a sensual, tender flame; a breath moving gently over your skin; kisses lingering in the hollow of your neck; little bites on your ear lobe, and naughty whispers. Nothing asked for and demanded beyond what is there for both of you in the moment. No other goal or pursuit or striving, no effort or labor. Slow Burn is not boredom, but something entirely different. A different kind of passion learned in confessional intimacy. A seasoned passion only a seasoned couple can achieve. A sensual

knowledge only you and she can know. Marriage is an excellent place for carnal knowledge.

Really, think about it...

TOOLKIT

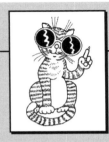

DO:

✓ Start to recognize the possibility of another kind of desire.

✓ Learn to know another kind of passion.

✓ Get curious about Slow Burn and experiment with it.

✓ Celebrate every step you make in this direction. (Slow Burn will last until death do you part.)

✓ Expect that in any long-term relationship some form of Hot-Burn-crisis will arise.

✓ Expect that one of you will fall in love with someone else, start flirting, be tempted and perhaps act out.

✓ Be prepared; it could be you.

✓ Imagine what it would take to come to complete, shared understanding.

✓ Consider the possibility of being forgiven.

✓ Realize that forgiveness and understanding are different names for the same thing.

✓ Consider this: the two of you might have a chance to begin all over again, both changed, more mature, more whole-hearted and loving.

DON'T:

✗ Don't be a fool and throw in the towel the minute things start to cool off.

✗ Don't blame your lover for things slowing down.

- ✗ Don't constantly remind her of how she used to be when you first met.

- ✗ Don't run out to look for the Hot Burn with someone else.

- ✗ Don't compare your relationship to all the wild affairs you've had before (which obviously never lasted).

- ✗ Don't compare your sexuality to your best friend's. (She just fell in love.)

- ✗ Don't brood; use a tool from the kit.

- ✗ Don't harp; play with the tools.

- ✗ Don't focus on what you don't have.

- ✗ Don't be a sex-perfectionist.

- ✗ Don't think good enough is less than good enough.

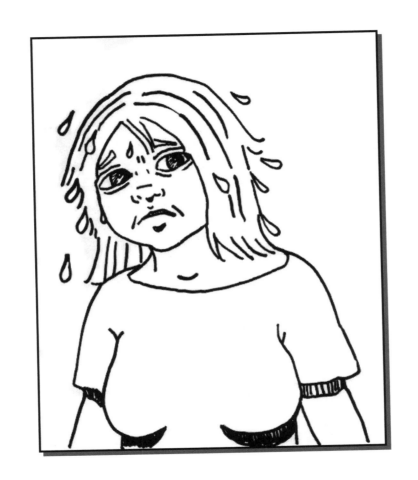

CHALLENGE 9

IN THE RING – FIGHTING FAIRLY

Written by Renate.

There is a couple I know. I've known them pretty well, for twenty-eight years to be exact (not counting the three and a half years of their friendship through letter writing and mutual editing exchanges.) After all this time of happy, inspired togetherness, this couple still fights. Should I be embarrassed about that? Not in the least. The fights Kim and I have now tend to go "puff!" and are gone. We shake our heads about them as they eternally repeat our basic temperamental differences. One of us usually spots the pattern and points it out. We now have well rehearsed ways out of the bad mood and anger of a discord or fight. As the years have gone by, we have become better at it. We've come a long way, baby.

Our first big fight happened after we had just fallen in love and spent three excited weeks in Paris and the south of France. Kim had returned to the States to attend her daughter's graduation.

On the phone, with a romantic tease in her voice, she asked: "So when do you come over here to marry me?" I was speechless. I didn't notice the humor. She already knew I was not the marrying kind. I had several lovers and was proud of my polygamous lifestyle.

My outrage over this proposition led to an angry exchange. Finally, Kim pointed out that she had been playing with Jewish humor: you say what is taboo, you spell out the forbidden thing, the hidden secret... and laugh about it. If you can. Not me. "We hardly know each other," I challenged her. "We might soon be like every other couple I know -- bored!" "There's one thing I can promise you," she said, "You'll never be bored with me." This cocky arrogance triggered me even more, and I made a long speech about not committing to anything before I had solid proof.

Well, the proof came with time. It came with a few rollercoaster years of bliss and passionate fights. I discovered that Kim was a hothead and an impeccable fighter with words and arguments. I rushed into therapy to get support. I complained to my therapist that I felt pushed against the wall because Kim was yelling in our fights.

"What's wrong with yelling?" she wanted to know. I was thrown by the simple curiosity in her question. My outrage collapsed in a second. What I was left with was the fact that I came from a family where nobody was supposed to raise their voices and disagreements were politely brushed under the carpet. This suddenly did not seem an advantage. "Fighting can be learned," my therapist mused, giving me something more to think about. When I told Kim about this unexpected reaction she said, "But you are, in fact, really good at it. Don't you know that?" I didn't, although I remembered wild fights with my sister as a child, so perhaps Kim was right. I could dare to stand up for myself and even yell back if I had to.

One topic of heated fights was my entanglement with my European lovers. I fiercely maintained my feminist lesbian right to keep every past lover close to my heart (and occasionally even in my bed). Love was not supposed to be possessive; love was about sharing. This drove Kim nuts, especially the way I would visit my old love pals in Europe and forget to call her and reassure her about what was going on.

Finally, my therapist again gave me food for thought. "It seems to me that Kim gives herself completely to this relationship," she said, "so there's an imbalance in the commitment." Once, in her exasperation, Kim had said to me, "You want to have it all, but you are hurting our relationship." It was clear I had to make a choice. I had to understand the reasons I could not let go of my exes in order to become an equally engaged partner with Kim.

LESBIAN MARRIAGE: A SEX SURVIVAL KIT

Like most couples, we had fights over money. Kim was an established, successful writer and counselor for women with eating disorders; I had always lived a bohemian lifestyle as a cultural journalist with lots of free time for creative projects. I now had to start over in a different language and culture. There was no financial equality in our relationship, quite the opposite. We were living Kim's lifestyle, not my old Parisian bohemian make-do-with-nothing.

We tried to deal with the challenge in different ways. A clear work division gave me house, garden, shopping, and cooking to take care of, and when I started making money as an editor and writer, we split our bills according to our earning potential -- Kim shouldering two thirds and I one third. But I still felt like the poor cousin who had to ask for many personal things I needed or desired. This was painful and sometimes humiliating --until I went back to school to become a therapist and then a spiritual counselor, building a solid foundation for my existence in the States.

In spite of our pervasive sense of being life companions with many compatibilities, the process of feeling equally empowered in our relationship took time. Eventually, it didn't matter any more who paid for how much and who paid more; we felt we were making the same amount of efforts; we were sharing everything; we were together for better or worse.

There are still topics that can get a rise out of us. We still quarrel, for example, when we are hosting friends. If four are coming to dinner, Kim shops for ten. She loves to load up the table as if there were no tomorrow, while I argue that this "overkill" of abundance is slightly sickening and worrisome because of the unnecessary expense. We recognize the clash between a Jewish culture of overflowing generosity (I would call it "let's eat what we can today as there might be a pogrom tomorrow ") and a German culture of post-war scarcity and noble restraint for the sake of savoring the smallest bits and bites as treasures.

The pattern is so deeply established in our temperaments, so second-nature, that we can slip back into a momentary discord faster than we can catch ourselves. "Who's going to eat all that food?" "Who cares? The point is to have it there. What kind of celebration can you have without enough food?" "Okay sure, enough for the entire neighborhood?" "So, when is enough ever enough?" But we do catch it. We decided that we would have gravestones next to each other with Kim's saying MORE and mine saying ENOUGH ALREADY.

LET'S SEE...

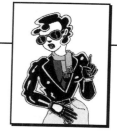

I have often tried to put my finger on the inner process I would go through that kept me from throwing in the towel and taking the next plane back to Paris. I could best describe it as turning my head right at the edge of the abyss to look back at her. I might have slammed a door to my room or run into the garden, tearing my hair out. Then, after a moment of breathing, a small voice would speak up in my heart. There was a mixture of sorrow and doubt.

What if there were a kernel of truth in her fiery accusation and reproach? What if my defensiveness was just a cover-up for my pride or for something unsavory I had done? After some time alone, listening to the storm inside me, I would discover how deeply it hurt me that my beloved, my life companion, was so wounded and upset...by me.

I sensed that when two lovers get into a passionate fight, there had to be a deeper truth, perhaps a sexual truth, that hasn't been found and hasn't been spoken. The way we fought was also the way we were as lovers. What troubled us as fighters delighted us as lovers. Kim's hot-headedness was a gift in bed; my cooler disposition an enticement to her to conquer me and melt the ice. For us, as for most other lovers we knew, sex was reborn after a fight, but wasn't a reason to fight.

Fighting always entails suffering; it requires an intense process of approaching each other again from our far-flung "hostile" positions. We discovered that there were small but crucial steps we could take without caving in, without giving up our sense of self, our truth, the sense of outrage and pain over whatever had led to the fight and escalated the outrage. I could go back to her with a trembling heart and say, "Maybe I am unfair and don't see your point. But I am sure you do have a point." The angry tension would instantly subside.

Kim would make a similar tiny step toward me. "That's all that matters to me, really. Just that you see I might have a point." Sometimes one of us could say, "Sorry for my part in this mess. Whatever it is I did badly, I regret it and want to understand it." Another big notch down. The familiar and beloved other would be recognizable again.

With more anger and fear cooling off, I would be able to say, "But I have a point, too, and I need you to hear me out and truly understand where I came from." Where I came from was not necessarily something to be proud of, but as we admitted our truth step by step, we always found that even a bitter confession would be enlightening to both of us.

In a shared spirit of fairness, we would come to a place of apology or simple acceptance because we had both been understood. If a problem is fully understood, forgiveness is a short step away. The problem, if it remained, would now be calmly and clearly visible, and, therefore, creative solutions could be found. Imagine a marriage where every fight leads to understanding, forgiveness, and healing.

TOOLKIT

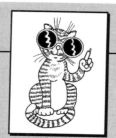

DO:

✓ **Gather a repertoire of simple things to say that prevent the escalation of fights:**

✓ *I'm sorry.*

✓ *Let's not go there.*

✓ *Let's be friends.*

✓ *We are still friends, aren't we?*

✓ *You have a point.*

✓ *We both have a point.*

✓ *Can you understand and forgive me?*

OTHER PRACTICES:

✓ Have a safe place.

✓ Go to it when you can't stop the escalation.

✓ Take time out, take time in.

✓ Catch the pattern and begin to see the humor.

✓ Laugh about it.

✓ Relish your fight if you have to have one and then make up.

✓ Use practiced formulas (like the repertoire above) for peace-making.

✓ Console each other for wounds inflicted.

✓ Correct blows below the belt.

✓ Clarify what you said but didn't really mean.

✓ Believe the one who says she didn't mean it.

✓ Apologize for your share in the fight.

✓ It always takes two to tango, so tango.

✓ Forgive.

DON'T:

✗ Don't perpetually think you are right; you can't be.

✗ Don't think that winning a fight does you any good.

✗ Don't think that any one fight will resolve all your differences.

✗ Don't go on all night.

✗ Don't use provocative language that enflames the fight. ("I'm out of here. I can't take this anymore. This is the absolute end of our relationship.")

× Don't leave without saying where you are going and how long you are taking time out.

× Don't forget that taking time out is different from slamming the door and walking out.

× Don't bring up issues more than six months old. (You know who you are.)

× Don't compare your lover to your ex.

× Don't divulge unresolved fights to your friends without prior agreement.

× Don't forget that curse words like: "you bitch, you slut, you whore, you dirty pig," are not exactly creative.

× Don't indulge in character assassination and humiliation. ("You've never been able to tell a single truth in your whole life. I can't see how anybody could ever have loved you. You are a failure from A to Z. You will never succeed in anything. You are the type of person who always... who never...")

× Don't allow the hostile echo of your own parents' voices to dominate a fight.

× Don't blame her for yelling when you are yelling, too.

× Don't underestimate your cold, quiet rage; its force is the equivalent of yelling.

× Don't imagine that the superior person is the one who never raises her voice.

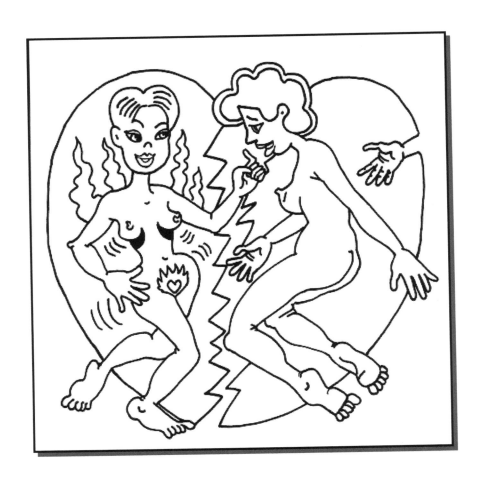

CHALLENGE 10

TO SEX OR NOT TO SEX

Kim's account of an extended monologue from a listening session.

FRANKIE: It's been this way since we first got together. We're not one of those couples who have this great erotic past to look back at. She's younger than I am, and all she ever wanted was extreme experience, to feel alive, and to have excitement. She couldn't lie down next to me and talk...that was too dull, too slow; it didn't take her out of herself. She wanted me to make her feel better about herself. She used to say, in this really miserable voice, "The only way I ever feel loved is when we make love. When you don't want to make love to me, I feel neglected and abandoned."

She'd never been in a relationship that had any peace or intimacy. She and her endless number of exes were always breaking off and getting together again. Splitting and making up, and that's what sex meant to her. Her idea of a good sexual relationship was, throw your lover on the floor and jump on top of her. I don't think she's ever, ever had a calm, intimate sexual experience in her life. So when that's what I wanted she'd be scornful and dismissive. Everything I did was wrong, turned her off instead of on.

She'd get furious and push me out of the bed. She'd start talking about breaking up with me. She'd lock the door to our room, and I wouldn't see her again until the next day. Then she'd slip onto the couch with me early in the morning and apologize, and I'd apologize for being such a klutz. We'd kiss and make up, but it sure wasn't sexual, and I didn't want it to be. Who'd want to go through all that again?

I kept saying, "Show me what you want, tell me what I should do. If I don't know how, teach me." But she'd say, "If I have to tell you, there's no excitement; the magic's gone; its just like you're following a blueprint." She'd tease me by calling me Madame Engineer, but I still don't think it's funny and that's where we still are.

I think she's too scared and inhibited to be intimate or tender. What she calls passion is really this huge rush to get it over with. I think no matter what I do, that's what it comes down to. But of course I'd never tell her that, or she'd accuse me of always blaming her. But really, when you come down to it, she's always blaming me.

So, here's the next funny thing. Most of the time, we're really happy together; you'd never believe we just can't get along when it comes to sex. I play the piano, and sometimes when we're in a good mood she'll start singing. Then we're dancing and she'll be humming, and the dogs come barking and everything's cool until we go to bed. So, I think, let's just stay up all night so we don't have to face this. Because it's always the same. We're excited, we're turned on, and then the whole thing crashes and we start to fight.

There's other times when it's not really about sex at all. It comes up when we're in some other kind of tension, something really dumb like who left the dishes in the sink. That's when she'll start shouting about how she can't go on without sex, and she's tired of supporting me, and I should damn well do the dishes because the money comes in from her. As if I don't work, which I do. But how is a second grade teacher supposed to compete with the millions she inherited from her grandmother even before she was out of college?

I'm perfectly happy to do the shopping and cooking. You wouldn't want to eat what she cooks anyway. She's never shopped or cooked in her life. If you send her out to get olive oil, she comes back with balsamic vinegar. She's miffed because it isn't the right thing, so I end up making a salad without oil. She tries to eat it just to show me we didn't need oil anyway, but of course we can't swallow the stuff. Right then, is when she's saying she can't go on without sex. But is it really about sex?

I mean, we have to straighten out all these other issues that are coming up, and we can't if sex gets mixed up in them, and we can't work on our sex life if we're trying to figure out who should do the dishes.

When I try to spell it out for her she says I always live in my head, and that's the problem with me. But what's so complicated about all this? Sometimes we fight because we don't know how to make love. Sometimes we don't fight, and we have a good time. Sometimes we say we're fighting about making love, but we're really fighting about the other issues we have.

I've proposed a moratorium on sex because that's the hardest for us to handle, and now we're both afraid if we agree to that, we'll never go back to having sex. I think, so what? Can't you have a really good relationship without it? You know that song... "Love and marriage, love and marriage / They go together like a horse and carriage. / Dad was told by Mother/ You can't have one without the other." Well, we certainly don't believe that anymore. So do we have to believe you can't have marriage without sex? Who says? Who made up that rule?

All the couples we know, and I mean all the heteros and a lot of the boys, too, are complaining about not having sex. So wouldn't we be better off if we all agreed, great, that's how it is; so let's concentrate on all the other ways of being close and getting pleasure and being excited? Take away the blame, you know. No one's to blame. That's just how it is, and what's wrong with that?

I can just imagine the relief that would go galloping into our lives if we all agreed to have all the sex we could before marriage, or when we wanted to have babies if you're that kind of couple, and that's it. We're done; we settle down into the next stage of life, and sex is just not part of it? And maybe that sex-free stage is what we call marriage.

Maybe we find some new names for the other stages like courting-sex or making-babies sex. But marriage has its own ways of being close and sex just doesn't have to be one of them. Why can't we just face the truth?

What does it tell us that after a few years the men go outside of marriage to have sex, and have a mistress or many mistresses or a prostitute in every port, or watch pornography, or go after the children in the family, or need Viagra? And the women? As one hetero said to me, "We women don't care about husbands anymore. We prefer our vibrators." So, my question is: why are we fighting this? Let's just look reality in the face and say, "Okay marriage, that's what you're like. I accept you."

LET'S SEE...

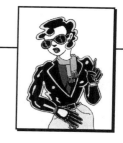

Shocking, isn't it? A woman thinking a thought that is virtually unthinkable in our sex-driven culture. Of course it's true that long-term relationships and marriage often face a gradual and perhaps indefinite cooling off of sexual heat. Maybe what we have humorously called "lesbian bed death" stands for a general condition? Maybe the label covers up an embarrassment that holds true for heterosexual and gay male couples as well? It's so convenient to make fun of a minority group for a majority condition, to imagine "they" have the problem and "we" do not. Yet, more often than not, long-term couples find they enjoy forms of closeness that don't involve sex. What's the problem? Why feel bad about not having something you no longer want?

This unthinkable thought asks us to think it.

Take travel, for instance. We remember wanting to go all over the world, see everything, meet everyone, have as much sex as possible. But after a dozen such trips, you begin to wonder about traveling. Vacations can be exhausting, expensive, repetitive, frustrating; you never get any further into a culture but remain outside looking in; you get a peek and not much real connection. But when the holidays are over and you didn't take a trip, your friends all have anecdotes and interminable photo displays, and you have nothing to say for yourself.

Since the word "staycation" came into use, we have pretty much understood that we enjoy staying home for our holidays, if only we didn't envy the people who go abroad.

Envy and competition, good old friends; social agents that act in our beds as well as in the marketplace. What a big role they play in the stories we tell, and the denial we practice about our sex lives. I've known people who feel so acutely the need to be part of an imagined sexual elite, they go after sex because it will make a good story. It reminds me of adolescent boys showing off how much sex they've had; it doesn't matter that their stories are often untrue and more compelling than the sex act itself, even for the testosterone-driven. Shall we face it? And if we face it, how about facing it with a wholehearted embrace? You're not alone. There's great comfort in being part of a gradually cooling 99%.

TOOLKIT

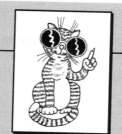

DO:

✓ Dare to think the unthinkable.

✓ Face a taboo.

✓ Question deprivation when there is none.

✓ Challenge cultural pressure.

✓ Examine your own relationship.

✓ Be rigorously honest about your desire for sex.

✓ If you are ambivalent, explore both sides of the coin.

✓ Read this book and discuss how to preserve sex if you want sex.

✓ Read the vibrator story.

✓ Consider that your cuddling may be sexual, after all.

✓ Question everything you've been taught to think about marriage and sex.

✓ Examine your assumptions.

✓ Appreciate and cultivate what already works in your relationship.

✓ Develop non-sexual, full-sensual pride.

✓ Be the rebel you are, if you are.

DON'T:

✗ Don't berate yourself and your partner for not wanting sex.

✗ Don't think your relationship isn't all it's supposed to be without sex.

- ✗ Don't compete in the sexual Olympics.

- ✗ Don't envy (or believe) your storyteller friends.

- ✗ Don't think that you are missing out on something everyone else has.

- ✗ Don't think sex is the only valuable form of sensual intimacy.

- ✗ Don't confuse sex with physical pleasure.

- ✗ Don't make sex the solution to your emotional problems.

Notes, Scribbles, Doodles

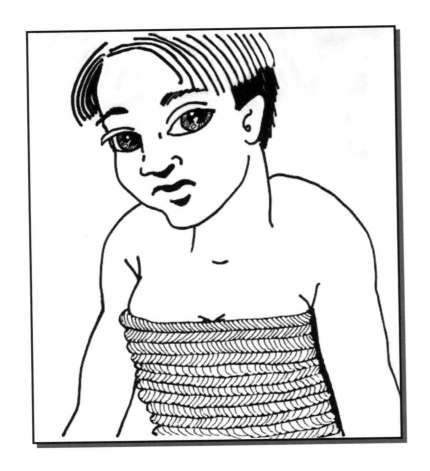

CHALLENGE 11

THE MAKE-OVER MARRIAGE — THOSE TRICKY EXPECTATIONS

Renate's account of a story told in a listening session.

CARLIE: I love her breasts! Why doesn't that make a difference? She has the most beautiful breasts, and she hates them. I'm happy with my big boobs but she, she doesn't want me to touch them anymore, and she binds them when we go out dancing. It hurts me to see those red straps over her squished flesh when I get a peek, but of course she does everything to not let me see. She keeps clothes on in bed, tight sports bras and tops, and it really bothers me, this cocoon she keeps herself in, keeping herself away from me. When we cuddle or spoon at night, I wrap my arm around her and feel the softness of her in a sneaky way. The rest of her is muscle, beautiful because she works it. She loves her rock climbing and being a wilderness guide, and she's a winner at that.

She won't talk about it. "We've said it all," is what she says every time, "why harp on it. I don't like my body; I hate my breasts, and I hate how they bump about on me like two sacks of fat, and I'm sure they are doing something malicious, breeding a cancer!" And I say, "Yeah the way you treat them, you're gonna trigger that." But I do understand, she is a boi person, and I am not. I said to her many times she could have a breast reduction; why not?

But that's not good enough for her, and it scares me. Because nothing's good enough for her about her body except her tattoos. And it's not that she thinks she's in the wrong body, not at all. She likes her down there. It's something else that eats her up. I think she feels she doesn't amount to much, at least compared to her high and mighty dad. But instead of dealing with that, like how she idealizes him, she talks about how she would do boxing if only her breasts weren't in the way!

I see her turning into a trans the moment I say, "Okay, go for it. I love you any way." But I'm not

126

sure it's true. It scares the shit out of me to think what will happen when she takes hormones and really starts the thing. Every time she goes to hang out with other trannies, I get nervous. Me? They despise me. I see their glances and little smirks, and I get mad. Well, she's not like that; she's really vulnerable inside, and I love that about her.

She confessed to me once that she's also scared of the testosterone. Her best friend from high school had a relationship with a girl who transitioned and became somebody she didn't even recognize any more, a guy with a beard and big pecs who started dating other men. It's eating her and if she had the money she would maybe just get rid of her breasts. And she might not stop there, why would she? It would still be eating her up, and she might want to go all the way with the hormones.

And that's the other problem. She says what would help her is my being on her side and not questioning her all the time. She says it would empower her if I really showed my trust and support by getting married. I thought about it a lot. We mostly have a great time together, although not sexually. We both work for Outward Bound, do our own wilderness trips, and we do catalogue design for a nature company. We're really creative together and that means a lot to me.

I haven't had a real relationship before, and neither has she. That's a big investment for both of us, and we can't imagine loving anyone else. So why not marry? But I know she'll get a big wedding gift from her parents who are big-shot liberals, and her mom has been active in the fight against Prop 8 to get gay marriage through the courts. So they are also putting pressure on us, and I'm pretty sure she will use the money to change that body of hers that I love so much. What then? What if I end up being married and not finding her a turn-on any more?

LET'S SEE...

RENATE: Marriage is not the remedy for couple trouble! But there is a lot of magical and wishful thinking about it: marriage will give you a new start, fix your problems, fulfill your dreams... It's the myth of the "Make-Over Marriage." (Should we call it MOM?) The romantic investment in marriage is huge. And so is the pressure. Couples trap each other with expectations, especially if some or all of their friends have already stepped up to the altar.

Who will pop the question? When will you pop the question? Are you saying our love isn't good enough? That I am good enough to be your partner but not your spouse? Prove to me that you love me by marrying me. Show me that you stand behind me and accept me with all my unsolved problems for better or worse.

Of course you want to begin again and be reborn a better person than you were a minute ago. Behind every oath and vow, there's a wish to rise again from your ashes. "I will love you forever" means I will become a person capable of loving forever; "until death do us part" means I am capable of sticking around for better or worse in an intimate relationship. "I give you my soul and my body" means I would like to be free of my sexual hang-ups. "With this ring, I thee wed" means I wish that our bond was stronger than all our differences and difficulties.

Marriage is a trickster. It's a new challenge for lesbian couples who might feel that now, as we may, we must.

TOOLKIT

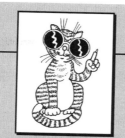

DO:

- ✓ Take marriage seriously and realistically.

- ✓ Be aware that institutions, even "sacred" ones like marriage, usually don't make people better.

- ✓ Be aware: marriage is not a guarantee for sex (and even less for sex ever-after.)

- ✓ Resist pressure, take your time, stay in the NOW of your relationship.

- ✓ Accept not being sure.

- ✓ Accept Not Yet.

- ✓ Be honest.

- ✓ Resist peer and family pressure.

- ✓ Resist your lover's need to prove anything through marriage.

- ✓ Open up your old copy of Women Who Love Too Much.

- ✓ Make up your own mind. (You will bear the consequences.)

- ✓ Weigh all the pros and cons before rushing to tie the knot. (It's better to break up over marriage now than suffer a divorce later.)

- ✓ Get advice from other married couples or marriage counselors.

- ✓ Consider consulting a property/tax attorney.

- ✓ Make sure you know about each other's credit card debts.

✓ Spell out any conditions without fear. Do it now. (Later is too late.)

✓ Remember that a good marriage isn't all that easy to pull off.

DON'T:

✗ Don't believe that marriage will fix your lover or her problems.

✗ Don't think that marriage will fix your own problems.

✗ Don't marry because you believe you'll miss out on the most romantic part of your relationship.

✗ Don't marry because it's the fashion right now.

✗ Don't marry because it's "a fun game," and you'll get lots of gifts.

✗ Don't rush because of the historical moment.

✗ Don't believe that marrying proves your love.

✗ Don't believe that marriage means you stand behind your lover for better or worse.

✗ Don't count on marriage to magically make love or sex deeper or better.

Notes, Scribbles, Doodles

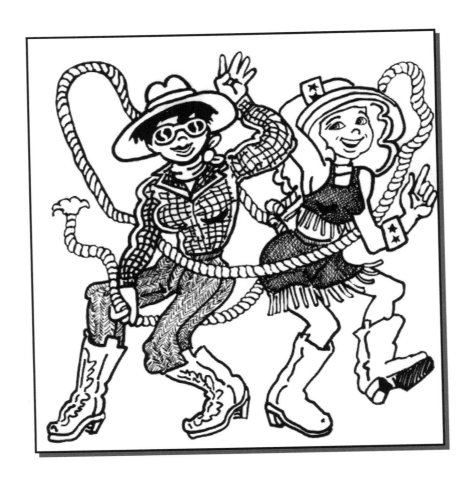

CHALLENGE 12

TYING THE KNOT — RE-INVENTING MARRIAGE

Kim's account of a story told by a young friend.

RIVKA: Of course, I want to get married. But I don't see why we have to rush down there the minute City Hall opens. She thinks we ought to go stand in line the night before, and I'm saying, like we're going to stand around all night long? So she's convinced I don't want to get married. And I'm saying I want us to do it our own way. Because if it's going to be romantic we sure don't want City Hall. And she's saying we can have City Hall and then have the romantic stuff at the beach or the zoo or somewhere. I never thought the Supreme Court was going to go for it. And she didn't either, so I thought we had plenty of time.

Now all of a sudden we're in this rush, and I don't like it. Our friends say I'm having trouble with commitment, and I'm saying, "Hey, you didn't have my mother, did you?" I always wanted to write a story about my mother. I'd call it: The Woman With Three Wives. One of these days I'll sit down and do it even if I have to wait until she and all the wives aren't around to read it.

When I was seven that's when they broke up. My mother and father banged doors and shouted, and she got her first wife. I'm not making fun of them by calling them wives. That's what she called them. She brought the first wife home and said, "This is your second mother." I was a smart ass so I said, "One mother's bad enough, now I have to have two of them?" My mother didn't like it, but the first wife did and she almost died laughing, so, of course, I started liking her.

She wasn't a wife at first because they hadn't had their ceremony. Ceremony was a big deal for Mom, and, pretty soon after she got a lot of money from my father, we had her big deal...okay, no need to describe it. Well, okay, why not? Just imagine a hundred people, most of them women. All dressed up and taking pictures and toasting everyone in sight with their pink champagne. I mean, like, even

CHALLENGE 12: TYING THE KNOT — RE-INVENTING MARRIAGE

the waiters. There was a chocolate fountain with real French chocolate and that's where I hung out, like I would have known the difference between French chocolate and a Mounds bar. But I gobbled so much chocolate, I've never taken one bite of it since.

Of course, Mom and first wife weren't legally married, but they were married in their own way which was good enough for Mom, until it wasn't. So, when I was almost ten I got my second second mother, and we had another big deal, but I was having a hard time because I missed my first second mother. But there she was in the wedding procession, and she didn't seem to mind one bit. By that time my dad was also in the procession with Harold, his new lover, so we were just one crazy party, very, very Berkeley. I said three wives, and that means three second mothers for me, who all hung out with us and celebrated birthdays and holidays and so on because that's how it is when wives marry wives and raise a child together.

Well, I'm not going to end up with a fucking Chocolate-Fountain-Wedding like Mom wants for me. She thinks now it will feel real because it's legal. She thinks her problem was how it wasn't ever legal and that's why all the marriages split up. She's on about Ellen and Portia, "See how things have worked out with Portia because it's legal?" She says I could have a white tux and I say like, are you kidding? I'd rather wear my Chinese cargo-pants.

My mom always confided in me, so after a while I noticed that whenever a new wife came on the scene my mom said exactly the same thing about her and offered the same reasons to get married. Like she was always marrying the same woman, with the same feelings. She always believed in the ceremony, the magic ceremony, I mean four times in a row (including my Dad). She went right on believing in the ceremony because sooner or later the ceremony would get it right, and the wives would stay with her forever.

I don't know if it will be different now because it's legal. What I know is I don't want any illusions when I get married and no big parties and no fooling myself that because we're married we'll never grow apart. My idea is we go to Peru, and we find a woman shaman and get her to marry us at Machu Picchu, and then we come back and hit City Hall. I mean, why does a honeymoon have to take place after a marriage? Who made up that rule? I want to look her straight in the eyes and say, heck I don't know if this will last forever but I love you, so I hope it will. I hope it will. That's a lot to put on the line with another person.

So, I guess yes, okay, I'm willing because I know it's going to make her happy. That's what I want no matter how many second mothers I've had and that's the best reason I can think of for getting married. But it can't just be the same old stuff, like two women together is just a copy of a man and woman together, which it is not. It can't be, so why should it be? Two women legally married together is something new in the world, and that makes us something new in the world.

So we better find some new meaning in it and some ceremony that says, like, we know this, we're aware of it, we're something new. So when we say, I give you my heart and soul, I give you my body, we don't mean what a woman means when she gives her body to a man. When she says that to a man, there's thousands of years of meaning in it, and a lot of bad stuff. Real bad old stuff. When women get married, it means a whole bunch of new things. Like, I'm giving my body to someone who cares about my pleasure. And that's not something you can take for granted, is it? You got that and you've got the whole bucket.

LET'S SEE...

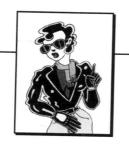

KIM: This is the voice of a very young woman. I am not a young woman, but I understand her demand that we do something new with the opportunity to marry. For some of us, legal marriage means that we are finally getting something men and women have had all along, to which we have a right. But there is also something else we're getting, if we want to take up the challenge. Rivka says: it's up to us to give a new meaning to an ancient ceremony that becomes new because two women are taking part in it.

The facts of marriage have changed repeatedly over time, and so, too, have the marriage-myths. Time for us to change them again and in our own terms. In an aristocratic marriage in the Middle Ages, there was never a question of romance, compatibility, or love; money and property met at the altar. The stereotypical model of the fifties, Mom and Dad and two kids, has diversified into blended, mixed-race, multi-generational, same-sex, and gender-queer families who sometime resemble tribes and often consist of one adult and one child. High time then to imagine marriage in our own pioneering spirit.

In spite of a great deal of talk about family values, traditional marriage is not exactly a successful institution. Half the people who get involved in it for the first time get back out again. The second time they try, sixty percent of them leave it behind.

It's also not the safest of institutions, when you consider that in 2009 (an average year) 24.2 % of murder victims were slain by a family member. 34.8% of female victims were slain by their husbands or boyfriends. In a recent statistic, 94% of child rape victims were abused by a family member. Among elder female victims who were abused, 78% suffered their assault from family members. Domestic violence is the leading cause of injury for women between the ages of 15 and 44. The family is a pretty dangerous place if you take these numbers seriously, as we should.

We are obviously not intending to make gay marriage a replica of conventional marriage with these serious dangers and this high incidence of abuse. So, what do we want? It's probably a good idea to have the discussion before we, and as we, and after we, rush down to stand in line all night at City Hall. There's no reason this conversation has to diminish our sense of celebration and joy. Why should it? It's here to remind us that we are involved in a historical moment that offers us the chance to become dreamers and visionaries.

We can revolutionize marriage to make it a happier, safer, more joyous place for ourselves and our kids. Remember, gay liberation and the struggle for women's rights will be standing right up there at the altar to give away the brides and grooms.

We've come a long way together...

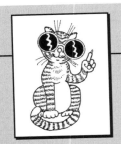

TOOLKIT

- ✓ **It's hard to see how tools could fashion a new vision of marriage. So, no more DO's and DON'Ts. Just one last tip:**

- ✓ **Start dreaming...**

EPILOGUE:

On October 28, 2013, Renate Stendhal and Kim Chernin had been together for 28 years. To celebrate, they got married.

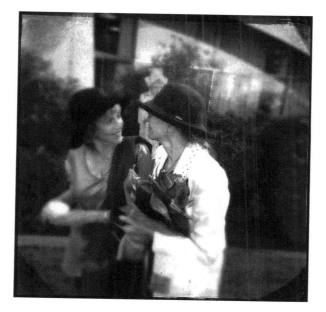

Photo: Louise Kollenbaum

RECEIVE A FREE ADDITION TO OUR TOOLKIT - OUR LESSONS IN EROTIC SPEECH

"SAY IT: THE DIRTY DOZEN"

Are you among those who approach love making like a lusty bear, pawing and grunting happily and not uttering a word? Are you the quiet type, fantasizing about steamy communication in bed, but too shy to speak? Would you like to have a few sexy words to turn your lover on? Our Dirty Dozen will give you ideas for things to say that are fun, hot, and sure to make an impact. Build up your repertoire of sexy communication.

Visit www.lesbiansexsurvival.com

www.kimchernin.com

www.renatestendhal.com

Notes, Scribbles, Doodles

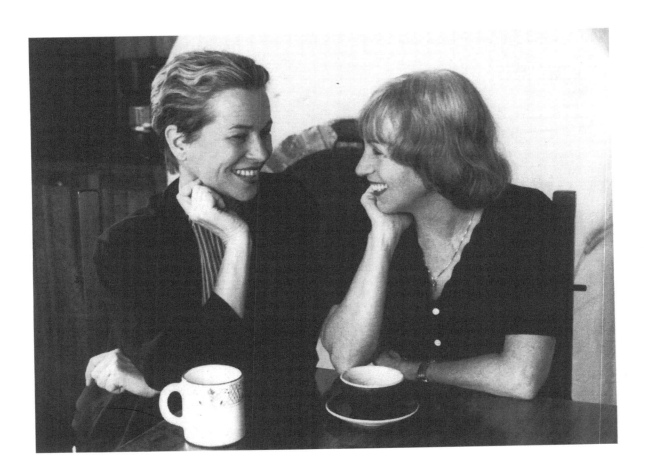

THE AUTHORS

Kim Chernin and Renate Stendhal are practitioners of a different kind of listening: a form of intuitive and common sense conversation. (Common sense because over the years we have realized that common sense is the least common kind of sense.) We have found that this type of conversation suits us and our clients better than therapy, counseling, or coaching. We invite our readers to continue the reflections presented here in a private, intimate setting. We are available to hold conversations with you individually or as a couple. Our offices are in the San Francisco Bay Area. Contact us through our websites:

www.kimchernin.com

www.renatestendhal.com

KIM CHERNIN

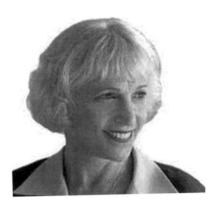

Kim Chernin's extensive body of work spans many genres, including fiction, nonfiction, memoir and poetry. Many of her seventeen published books are concerned with feminist and Jewish themes. Her book, *In My Mother's House* (1982) is regarded as a precursor of women's memoir writing. A number of her books are autobiographical, in particular *My Life as a Boy,* a coming-out story. She is an expert on women's relation to food and eating, author of the national bestseller *The Hungry Self.*

Kim and Renate have previously co-written *Sex and Other Sacred Games* and *Cecilia Bartoli: The Passion of Song.*

www.kimchernin.com

RENATE STENDHAL

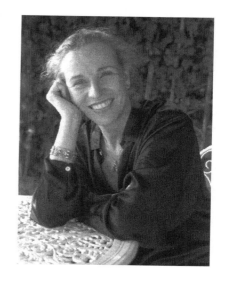

Photo: Cynthia Taylor

Renate Stendhal, Ph.D. is a German-born, Paris-educated writer and writing coach. She serves as provost, mentor, and practitioner of intuitive

listening and common sense conversation. She
has written several books, among them the award-
winning photo-biography, *Gertrude Stein: In Words
and Pictures,* which evolved into a Gertrude Stein
blog, "Why Do Something if it Can Be Done." Her
articles and essays have appeared internationally.
She is a senior cultural correspondent for the
international magazine for arts and media, Scene4.
She is working on an erotic Paris memoir.

www.renatestendhal.com

www.quotinggertrudestein.com

http://scene4.com/sc4bpaeo/stendhal.htm

http://www.huffingtonpost.com/
renate-stendhal-phd/

ACKNOWLEDGMENTS

Kim and I are old-school published authors. Before the revolution of e-books and books on demand we published many books in the traditional way, some of them award-winning and best-selling. We were curious about DIYS publishing, eager to experience the creative freedom and speed of this new publishing world.

Our adventure started with the First Self-Publishing Summit in Berkeley, in 2013, a weekend organized by She Writes publisher Brooke Warner (brooke@shewritespress.com) and Kindle expert Howard VanEs (Howard@letswritebooks.net.) I've been a member of She Writes for several years and started my Gertrude Stein blog for this community of women writers (quotinggertrudestein.com).

I attended the Summit as a journalist to explore and report from the electronic frontline of publishing (http://www.scene4.com/archivesqv6/jul-2013/0713/renatestendhal0713.html). Therefore, our first thanks go to Brooke and her pioneering Summit where I met Howard and got inspired by the promise of taking the publishing process in my own hands… with guidance. Expert guidance, as it turned out.

Howard VanEs amazed us with his keen sense for books in today's market, his caring attention to detail, his patience and great sense of humor. Working with Howard made it all seem fun from day one. Create a database? Start blogging and twittering? Create small YouTube videos? Help was needed and help arrived as Howard encouraged us to take charge of our book.

We had basically written our toolkit on vacation, house-sitting on Maui. Part of the time we were lying on the beach or haunting the beach cafés with our I-Pads. Sometimes we were like two cooks at the stove throwing bits of sentences into the same pot, together with good chunks of laughter. So much of our life experience, our own relationship, our work with clients got into the book because there was no censorship from a Publisher. We knew that our readers, our friends, would tell us what we needed to know. And they did.

Laura Stokes and Amy Schliftman in our West Marin neighborhood brainstormed with us before sending us off to Maui. Laura supplied us with a superb chapter-by-chapter analysis of an early draft, helping us focus and clarify our ideas. Gail Reitano and Joan Gelfand discussed the book with us and gave us poignant feedback. Joan said, "It only took a few thousand years to get to a book like this." Gail commented, "I can't see this confined to lesbian couples... everything you say pertains to being human."

Deborah Kory pointed out just in time everything that was still missing, and Lise Weil joked, "Marriage would have taken me less by surprise had I got an earlier peek ..." Our friends Jim van Buskirk and Leonard Cetrangolo added encouragement and good advice. VAs (Virtual Assistants in the brave new world of e-publishing) Kristen Reyes and Nicolas Sherman were a much needed and appreciated support. We felt lucky to be held by such a caring network of friends – not always, not only, maybe never, *lesbianistas*.

The creative freedom of independent publishing is like no other. We discovered this anew when we got to the book design, title and cover decisions. In traditional publishing you usually have to go to battle for your title and cover. We didn't have to fight with anyone.

Freedom opens the door to magic: Joey Hachtman (3dwstudios@omcast.net), cartoonist extraordinaire, came to us through Gertrude Stein. Let me explain. Tom Hachtman, equally brilliant cartoonist (gertrudefollies.com), had leant me his illustrations for my Gertrude Stein blog. Getting wind of our new lesbian toolkit, Tom sent along a sexy cartoon girl in leather, wearing shades and lipstick. This girl, it turned out, was a creation by Joey, his life companion. Kim and I fell in love with the naughty girl and instantly saw her on our cover. We told Tom, who told Joey, who read the manuscript and came back with a cornucopia of sketches. Another delicious, zany process of back-and-forth creation took place. One image really is worth ten thousand words.

Last, but not least, gratitude for our daughter's high spirits. Our wedding, which took place as soon as we finished the book, cracked her up. "What a relief," she said, "that you are finally not living in sin."

ABOUT THE ILLUSTRATOR

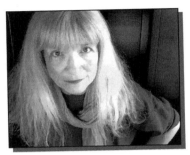

Joey Hachtman, illustration and cover design
Three Designing Women Studios: www.3dws.org

Long checkered career in art....painting, illustrating, cartooning, underground and above, animation, art direction, assisted Broadway set designer, and for the last nearly 20 years beautifying homes and businesses as a muralist.

Atheist, liberal...I lean so far left, I'm lying down!

Under my Twilight Zone High School yearbook picture it says I'd like to be remembered for not being a bigot! Still not!

Special thanks to partner T. Hachtman for helping color!

And to Myrna Lamb and Gertrude Stein for their contributions to the circle of life!

SELECTIVE BOOK LIST FOR KIM CHERNIN

All of the following books are available at your local bookstore and on Amazon.

MY LIFE AS A BOY: A WOMAN'S STORY

A young woman leaves her marriage and falls in love with a woman. She pursues the object of her desire like a boy.

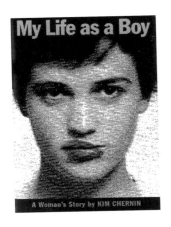

IN MY MOTHER'S HOUSE: A MEMOIR

A precursor of women's memoir writing, this story spans four generations of Jewish women in Chernin's family. The central character is Kim's mother, an immigration advocate who went to prison for her belief in justice.

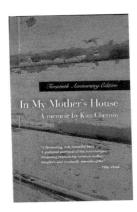

THE OBSESSION: REFLECTIONS ON THE TYRANNY OF SLENDERNESS

First part of a trilogy. Chernin, a pioneer in the field of eating disorders, places her own troubled relationship with food in a cultural context.

THE HUNGRY SELF: WOMEN, EATING, AND IDENTITY

Second part of the trilogy on women and food. Chernin explores the way women's craving for food is a longing for a larger female identity.

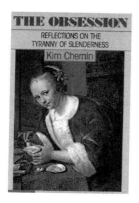

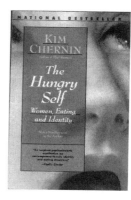

REINVENTING EVE: MODERN WOMAN IN SEARCH OF HERSELF

Third part of the trilogy on women and food. The taboo against eating the apple in the Garden of Eden is revealed as a prohibition against women's spiritual and personal development.

A DIFFERENT KIND OF LISTENING: MY PSYCHOANALYSIS AND ITS SHADOW

Chernin develops her own kind of intuitive listening as she presents her years on the couch with three renowned analysts.

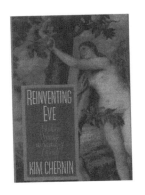

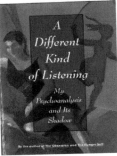

SELECTIVE BOOK LIST FOR RENATE STENDHAL

All of the following books are available at your local bookstore and on Amazon.

TRUE SECRETS OF LESBIAN DESIRE: KEEPING SEX ALIVE IN LONG-TERM RELATIONSHIPS

Foreword by Jewelle Gomez and new introduction by Renate Stendhal

Do you want your relationship to stay hot? The author reveals that telling the truth can be the healthiest, least costly, most effective aphrodisiac.

GERTRUDE STEIN: IN WORDS AND PICTURES

(with 365 photos by famous and unknown photographers)

A playful approach to the controversial genius, illustrating her life with photos, her best anecdotes and funniest one- liners, to show how approachable, fun, and even easy to understand Stein can be.

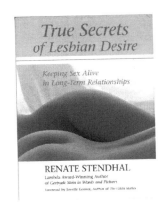

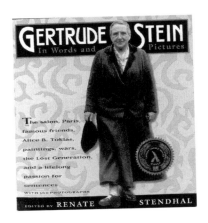

THE GRASSHOPPER'S SECRET: A MAGICAL TALE

(Illustrated by the author)

Available at Amazon. Read a sample of this book at http://tiny.cc/r5hx8w

A wisdom tale for children of all ages. Let a magical grasshopper take you on a time travel to Venice, Italy, where the suspenseful destiny of two kids unfolds.

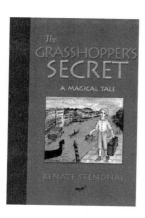

Notes, Scribbles, Doodles

BOOKS CO-AUTHORED BY KIM CHERNIN AND RENATE STENDHAL

All of the following books are available at your local bookstore and on Amazon.

CECILIA BARTOLI: THE PASSION OF SONG

The ten first years of the diva's world career described in detail: the only existing biography of this contemporary phenomenon of the opera stage.

SEX AND OTHER SACRED GAMES: LOVE, DESIRE, PASSION, AND POSSESSION

Two women meet in a Paris café and start a hot debate about love and sex. Their challenge to one another turns into a passionate relationship.

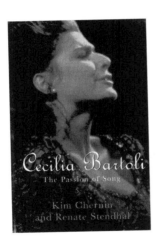

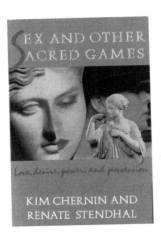

Made in the USA
San Bernardino, CA
07 June 2014